Gerald Schoenewolf, PhD

Psychotherapy
with People in the Arts
Nurturing Creativity

Pre-publication
REVIEW

"**P**sychotherapy with People in the Arts: Nurturing Creativity is a very readable and erudite treatise on the vicissitudes of the creative process and the potential relief provided to artists in conflict through therapy. In the rich and varied case studies, Dr. Schoenewolf carefully weaves the theoretical concepts of psychoanalytic thought with the concrete data of the tortured lives of his patients. The result is a stimulating and creative understanding of the artists' resistance to success and the resolutions of the neurotic behavior through interpretation.

This book is clearly an addition to the body of knowledge in the field and is of interest to both the professional and lay reader. The work will reaffirm the therapist's perception of neurotic behavior as symbolic and treatable. The lay reader will be fascinated to read about how the collaboration of patient and doctor to unravel the `layers of the onion' can restore the artist's creative functioning to its full potential."

Robert Pepper, PhD
Psychotherapist,
Forest Hills, NY

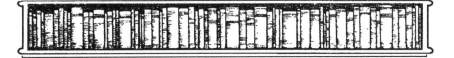

Psychotherapy
with People in the Arts
Nurturing Creativity

HAWORTH Marriage and the Family
Terry S. Trepper, PhD
Executive Editor

Psychotherapy
with People in the Arts
Nurturing Creativity

Gerald Schoenewolf, PhD

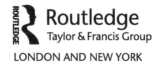

Routledge
Taylor & Francis Group

LONDON AND NEW YORK

First published 2002 by The Haworth Clinical Practice Press.

2 Park Square, Milton Park, Abingdon, Oxfordshire OX14 4RN
605 Third Avenue, New York, NY 10017

Routledge is an imprint of the Taylor & Francis Group, an informa business

First issued in hardback 2020

PUBLISHER'S NOTE
Identities and circumstances of individuals discussed in this book have been changed to protect confidentiality. Any resemblance to actual persons, living or dead, is entirely coincidental.

Cover design by Marylouise E. Doyle.

Library of Congress Cataloging-in-Publication Data

Schoenewolf, Gerald.
    Psychotherapy with people in the arts : nurturing creativity / Gerald Schoenewolf.
        p.   cm.
    Includes bibliographical references and index.
    ISBN 0-7890-1490-4 (alk. paper)—ISBN 0-7890-1491-2 (alk. paper)
    1. Artists—Mental health. 2. Psychotherapy—Case studies. 3. Creative ability. 4. Personality and creative ability.

RC451.4.A7 S36 2002
616.89'14'0887—dc21

2001039108

ISBN 978-0-7890-1490-0 (hbk)

CONTENTS

ABOUT THE AUTHOR

Gerald Schoenewolf, PhD, is Director of The Living Center in New York City, a cooperative of therapists who specialize in working with people in the arts. The center was founded in 1979. He is also Adjunct Professor of Psychology at Hunter College and at the New York Institute of Technology. He is a member of the American Psychological Association and the National Association for the Advancement of Psychoanalysis. Dr. Schoenewolf is the author of twelve books. Visit his Web site at <http://www.livingcenter.net>.

Preface

According to legend, F. Scott Fitzgerald once said to Ernest Hemingway, "The rich are different from you and me." To which Hemingway replied, "Yes, they have more money." One could say, however, that F. Scott Fitzgerald, Ernest Hemingway, and other creative people *are* different from you and me. People in the arts have a sensitivity that others do not have. That sensitivity makes them more attuned to all of the arts, providing them with an ear for music, an eye for color and design, and a mind that sees into the depths; that sensitivity may also make them more susceptible to certain emotional disorders.

The past several decades has seen the development of a special field of psychotherapy devoted to the treatment of artists. I have been one of those who helped to develop it. As Director of The Living Center in New York City for over twenty years, I have come up with my own way of working with people in the arts, using an eclectic approach that combines psychoanalysis, Gestalt therapy, psychodrama, behavioral therapy, art therapy, and meditation. The goal of the therapy is to free up artists from the emotional blocks that hamper them as artists and as people.

However, *Psychotherapy with People in the Arts* is not just a book on technique but also a book of narratives that allows readers to get an in-depth view of how various writers, artists, composers, and other creative people have coped with inhibitions in the creative process, rejection, fame, dysfunctional families, addictions, compulsions, and a host of other problems. It begins with an introduction that looks at the relationship between emotional disorders and creativity, focusing on the writer J. D. Salinger. It then continues with chapters about selected people in the arts with whom I have worked, showing the interrelation between their creative processes, their past lives, their present lives, and what goes on in the therapy office. Finally, there is an appendix with four tests that can be used to measure a person's inhibition of creativity.

My hope is that this work will be an inspiration to both professionals in the field and to artists—or indeed to all those who wish to enhance their creativity.

Acknowledgments

This book could not have been written without the artists, writers, and performers who were the subjects of its chapters. Although none of the case histories is based on any one person—each is an amalgamation of several people who had similar personalities and issues—they are nevertheless representative of those patients who were lucky enough to admit that they needed help and to be able to work through their creative blocks and achieve some success in both art and life. I thank them for allowing their stories to be used as examples in this book.

Chapter 1

The Cracked Mirror: Neurosis and Creativity

A debate has rattled inside and outside the halls of psychology: Do artists have to be neurotic? Is their neurosis essential to the production of art?

There are several schools of thought on the matter: One has it that artists are the sanest folks around, wielding a prophetic madness, possessed of a wisdom not shared by ordinary people. Another says that artists have special problems, are prone to particular kinds of mental disorders, and require a special kind of psychotherapy. A third contends that the special problems of artists contribute to their art and must not be tampered with by therapists. Another view maintains that artists needn't suffer and that neurotic suffering adversely affects their productions, causing them to create distorted art that likewise adversely affects society. Yet another argues that art and suffering go hand-in-hand, and that neurosis makes art more interesting and is beneficial to society.

From the beginning, most mental health professionals aligned themselves with those artists who saw suffering as part of the territory of creativity, contending that neurosis is essential to art. Sigmund Freud (1907) started this trend by linking creativity with one of his neurotic defense mechanisms. He believed that creativity was the outcome of sublimation; artists, writers, musicians, and other creative people are able to divert psychological conflicts and frustrations (such as frustrations in love) into some kind of creative enterprise. He observed that the desire for fame, power, and women lay behind the motivation to create. Hence, Freud believed that creativity was a compensatory function, not an original impulse.

1

Elsewhere he explains art as a turning away from reality:

> An artist is originally a man who turns away from reality because he cannot come to terms with the renunciation of instinctual satisfaction which it at first demands, and who allows his erotic and ambitious wishes full play in the life of fantasy. He finds his way back to reality, however, from this world of fantasy by making use of special gifts to mould his fantasies into truths of a certain kind, which are valued by men as precious reflections of reality. (1911, p. 244)

In a study of Leonardo da Vinci, Freud (1910) demonstrated that works of art could be analyzed like dreams and fantasies. He believed, for example, that the ambiguity in the smile of the *Mona Lisa* and other figures was the result of condensation stemming from the artist's unconscious conflicts about his mother. "In his madonnas he did not express the direct continuation of the mother's love but rather the defensive denial of her lack of love" (p. 81). Although da Vinci intended to paint loving madonnas, his unconscious conflicts about his mother and all women crept into his works so that the smiles were marked by ambivalence. Yet, while analyzing their products, Freud nevertheless viewed artists in a very positive light, claiming that creative writers were valuable allies of psychoanalysis since they were more in touch with their unconscious than social scientists. Their works were to be highly prized for "they are apt to know a whole host of things between heaven and earth of which our philosophy has not yet let us dream" (1907, p. 8). He added that their knowledge of the mind was far advanced from "us everyday people," despite whatever neurotic conflicts they had.

Other psychoanalysts have continued the debate. Rank (1932) looked at two aspects of creativity: he saw works of art as representing the artist's ego ideal and serving a reparative function. According to his theory, an artistic endeavor is the artist's attempt to transcend both his or her genetics and environmental conditioning to achieve a kind of heroism. Nevertheless, neurosis is central to Rank's concept: "Hardly any productive work gets through without morbid crises of a 'neurotic' nature" (p. 310). Kris (1952) coined the phrase "regression in the service of the ego," meaning that an artist is able to become a child or an idiot-savant in order to produce art. He explained that "We may speak here of a shift in psychic level, consisting in the fluctuation of a functional regression and control" (p. 253). Although, similar to Rank, he wrote of art and artists in an almost idealizing way, he nevertheless still linked the creative process with sublimation and attributed to it a reparative function. Rose, building on the work of Kris, notes that "Aesthetic experience is regarded as essentially a regression of one kind or another and aesthetic form primarily a defense against content" (1980, p. 8).

Alexander succinctly restates another familiar theme with regard to artists and creativity: that works of art can be analyzed like dreams in order to explore the artist's inner world. "Like dreams or daydreams, works of literature, painting, and sculpture are products of the creative fantasy which reflect the psychology of the artist" (1953, p. 346). Philips, going a step further, contends, "Neurosis, though not sufficient for the production of art, may be necessary for it" (1957, p. xvii). Writing about one particular German writer, Philips describes the writer as having a "neurotic predisposition toward ideas" (p. xviii).

Greenacre (1971) emphasizes the family romance in the lives and works of artists. This fantasy, in which the artist replaces his real parents (who are found lacking) with ideal ones, is created in order to defend against an excessive attachment to the parents in the postoedipal stage, to punish them for their sexuality (from which he feels left out), and to return to the relatively conflict-free days of the preoedipal period. Greenacre points out that family romances and related fantasies seem to predominate in the minds and artistic themes of artists.

Ludwig (1996) did a comparative study of emotional disturbances among artists and nonartists and showed that they were far more common among artists. He found, for example, that 60 percent of actors and 41 percent of novelists were alcoholics. However, only 3 percent of scientists and 10 percent of military officers were alcoholics. Likewise, 17 percent of actors and 13 percent of poets suffered from manic depression, while only 1 percent of scientists did so. Goodwin and Jamison (1990) uncovered impressive evidence of a link between creativity and manic depression. The list includes the writers Gertrude Stein, Virginia Woolf, Fyodor Dostoyevsky, William Shakespeare, Pablo Picasso, Tennessee Williams, Ernest Hemingway, William Styron, F. Scott Fitzgerald, Herman Melville, Eugene O'Neill, Henry James, and Honoré de Balzac; composers Robert Shuman, Hector Berlioz, and George Frideric Handel (who wrote *The Messiah* in twenty-four days during a manic high); artists Vincent van Gogh and Salvador Dalí; and the poets Poe, Tennyson, Byron, Shelley, and Coleridge. The implication is that manic depression—or bipolar disorder, as it is now called—is an essential ingredient of art, one that perhaps gives it vitality.

Niederland (1967) links creativity with depression, detailing a relationship between creative activity and reparative efforts after loss. He posits a permanent and usually severe injury to infantile narcissism of artists, giving rise to a relentless but futile struggle to recover from this loss. To back up his theory, Niederland lists numerous artists, poets, and composers who suffered serious injuries, defects, or illnesses, including Byron, Keats, Chopin, Toulouse-Lautrec, Mozart, and Hugo.

Bergler (1945), perhaps epitomizing what happens when classical psychoanalysis is taken to extremes of depth psychology, interprets five layers of the psyche of Leonardo da Vinci (taking as his starting point Freud's previous study of the artist). In the first layer there is regression in response to an id wish; in the second, this conflict is counteracted by a reproach from the superego; in the third, a defense mechanism is established; in the fourth, the defense mechanism is reproved by the superego; and finally, in the fifth, the ego sublimates, establishing a secondary defense or a defense against a defense. He concludes, "What is sublimated is neither the id wish nor the defense against the id wish but the defense against the defense against a conflict originating historically in an id wish" (p. 97).

Although the theme of art as a consequence of neurosis has been predominant and ongoing in psychoanalysis, another trend has also made its way into the literature. Writing about literary works, Bonaparte notes that the least neurotic works are the most objective, while those that are laden with the creator's complexes are most subjective. "At one extreme, we should find the writings of a Maupassant or Zola, works written almost impersonally. . . . In the latter [other extreme] the author's complexes, more or less masked, project themselves into the work" (1949, p. 55). This view suggests that neurosis mars creativity.

As previously noted, Greenacre (1971) looked at the family romance as a strong factor in the lives of artists, but she also saw innate endowment as the primary source of the creative process. She notes that there are serious limitations to the view of art as a product of psychopathology, since there are many works of art in which there is no evidence of psychopathology. Her theory is that artists possess a "predisposition to an empathy of wider range and deeper vibration" (p. 485), which lies at the root of their creativity.

Having specialized in working with people in the arts for over twenty years, I have also come to disagree with the notion that artists must suffer and their suffering (their neurosis, psychosis, personality disorder) is required for their creativity. Emotional disturbances do not enhance art. They may make it interesting, especially to that segment of their audience which suffers from similar disturbances. More often, disturbances cause artists to become blocked, unable to create or able to create somewhat distorted works. Ultimately, when we resolve disturbances and their underlying conflicts in therapy, we not only diminish the blocks but also increase the flexibility and objectivity of the artist so that the works produced have a more universal appeal. Art that is objective is, I would contend, more beneficial to society, since it points out the truth of the human condition.

Artists have always been important to society because of their impact on culture and their articulation of cultural values. As Shakespeare put it, the job of the artist is to "hold the mirror to nature." If the mirror is true, the insight is true. But if the mirror is cracked—if the artist suffers from a disorder that bends his or her view—then the insight will be more or less untrue. Psychoanalysis can help to clear up the distortions, provided, of course, that the psychoanalyst himself or herself does not also suffer from some kind of distortion of vision. As the writer Sidney Offit noted, "Although we may never entirely resolve the mysteries, art and psychoanalysts are our most constructive illuminations" (1998, p. 2).

Creativity would seem to be influenced by both nature and nurture. An apple tree is genetically programmed to produce a certain number of apples, but whether or not it produces those apples also depends on whether it receives adequate sunshine, carbon dioxide, and minerals and is protected from the elements. A gifted artist is perhaps genetically programmed to produce a certain number of works of art, but whether or not he or she does so depends on whether he or she receives adequate security, encouragement, acceptance, love, respect, and other intangibles as a child.

Many have argued that emotional trauma brings about the need for self-expression as a reparative measure. However, my own research convinces me that the reverse happens. It would appear that artists have a temperamental predisposition to develop certain disorders; in other words, their innate talent not only genetically programs them to produce works of art, but also makes them susceptible, due to a greater sensitivity to environmental conditions and a tendency to respond to those conditions through the development of manic-depressive, depressive, narcissistic, and masochistic features. And to the extent they develop any combination of these disorders, to that same extent their development affects their creative productions.

A case in point is the American writer J. D. Salinger. Although we don't have enough information about his childhood to determine the nature of his psychological development, due in part to the author's own much-noted secrecy, it would seem, based on his writings and from what little we do know about his life, that he suffered from one or more conditions. These disorders appear not only to have limited his productivity (he only published four short books of fiction), but also to have shaped the content of his writing in ways that impacted the universality of his perspective.

Salinger was born in 1919 in New York City. His father was a Jewish importer who became increasingly prosperous. His mother was Scotch-Irish. He had an older sister. The family moved several times during his childhood and finally settled into an apartment on East 91st Street (near where Holden Caulfield's family lived in his novel *The Catcher in the Rye*). Salinger was asked to leave two or three prep schools before his father finally sent him to the Valley Forge Military Academy, from which he graduated after two years. Holden Caulfield was on the verge of flunking out of Pencey, which may have been modeled after one of the prep schools he attended.

The first version of *The Catcher in the Rye* was a long story called "I'm Crazy," published in *Collier's* magazine. In this first version, Holden Caulfield is depicted as having problems at school due to pressures from his upwardly mobile parents. Later, in the final version of this story, *The Catcher in the Rye,* Holden's problems are not due to his parents but to the "phonies" who permeate society. This theme of the pure soul done in by the phonies of the world runs through Salinger's works. If we analyze these two versions of the story as we would the manifest content and secondary elaboration of a dream, we can see the secondary elaboration at work in the second version (the desire to protect the parents). We can also see in the second version the work of the ego ideal—the shift in his view of his protagonist (in whom he projects his self) from the "confused" boy in the first story to the adolescent savant who in fact is less confused than everybody else.

After graduating from the Valley Forge Military Academy, Salinger attended three colleges, including New York University and Columbia, but did not obtain a degree from any of them. He served in the army from 1939 to 1945, participating in the D day landing in France, and afterward was treated for combat-related stress. His story "For Esme, with Love and Squalor" touches on his war experience, telling the story of Sergeant X, who suffers from shell shock. After the war, Salinger began to write full-time and to sell stories to popular magazines.

The fiction in his four books was written during a twelve-year period, from 1951 to 1963. These included the one novel and three books of stories: *Nine Stories; Franny and Zooey;* and *Raise High the Roof Beam, Carpenters and Seymour: An Introduction.* He published two other stories, "Hapworth 16, 1924," which appeared in *The New Yorker* in 1965, and "Go Tell Eddie," which was part of an academic anthology in 1969. After these stories, Salinger never published again. He has reportedly been married and divorced twice and has two children by his second marriage. He has lived as a recluse in Connecticut and contends, in those rare moments when he has publicly spoken, to no longer care about fame or fortune.

Without looking at the content of his writings, it seems evident that his retreat from the world and the termination of his publishing activity when he was just at his prime signals the work of some underlying psychological conflict. His public statements to the effect that he is no longer interested in fame or fortune and has, instead, taken a Zen Buddhist path away from attachment to worldly ways, do not quite explain this shift. Rather, his abrupt retreat seems indicative of a narcissistic withdrawal from the impure world of phonies—a withdrawal, so it would appear, into a very private world of purity and higher consciousness.

One can see a trend in his fiction from his earliest work to his latest, a trend of progressive narcissism. In *The Catcher in the Rye,* the author heralds the theme of the pure soul corrupted by a corrupt world who, as I pointed out previously, might be seen as a fictional manifestation of the author's ego ideal, designed to compensate for the author's feelings of low self-esteem. Another theme of the work, the protagonist's tendency to get into situations in which he provokes punishment, such as in the first scene with the condescending elderly teacher, the encounter with the sadistic prostitute and her pimp, and the scenes with the verbally abusive cab drivers, would seem to demonstrate a masochistic feature of his personality. One also finds much depressive ideology in Holden's constant self-negation and sense of futility.

These themes are repeated, and become more exaggerated, in subsequent stories. In "A Perfect Day for Bananafish," Seymour Glass is the pure soul and his wife and her mother are the phonies who are driving him crazy. At the end of the story, he commits suicide. In "Franny," it is Franny Glass (one of seven Glass children) who plays the part of the pure soul, and her boyfriend, a snobbish boor of a young man named Lane, is the phony from whom she makes an abrupt run to the bathroom, where she sobs and reads a book of Eastern philosophy which Lane had disparaged. At the end of this story, Lane also proves to be a letch, interested only in getting her to go to bed with him. (In Salinger's works, it appears that only phonies want sex.) In "Zooey," the author fondly depicts several members of the Glass family, including Franny, her brother Zooey, and their mother, narrating the tale from the voice of their novelist brother, Buddy. This time, all three—as well as other Glass family members who are mentioned in passing—serve as projections of the author's ego ideal. In addition, there is a family flavor in this story that corroborates Greenacre's thesis about the importance of the family romance in the lives and works of writers. It is more clear than ever in this work that Salinger has concocted an ideal family which, according to Greenacre's thesis, is meant to replace his real family, punish them for their sexuality, and return him to a preoedipal period of conflict-free living. Indeed, a preoedipal innocence runs through not only this story but through all of Salinger's works; there are no positively portrayed sexual scenes in any of them, and sexuality is more often seen as lascivious, as it was in "Franny." The author attempts to depict the Glass family as spiritual people, uninterested in worldly matters; however, the case is made, again and again, that family members are not just spiritually above the rest, but also intellectually superior. Indeed, they are presented as a family of quiz kids, geniuses, and seers who know but do not tell what they know.

The theme widens and thickens in "Raise High the Roof Beam, Carpenters" and "Seymour: An Introduction." In both these stories, Seymour is the protagonist. In the former, he doesn't show up on his wedding day, presumably because of his purity and apparent awareness of the phoniness of his future wife and of the tainted (oedipally incestuous) convention of marriage. The latter story is a backward glance at Seymour, by Buddy Glass. By now Seymour has become idealized to the point of sainthood, and the rambling novella has no real plot, consisting simply of memories written with the reverence of the Gospel according to St. John.

In his last *New Yorker* story, "Hapworth 16, 1924," Seymour is presented as not just a saint, but as a veritable reincarnation of Buddha. The story, once again long, rambling, and plotless, is a letter written by a five-year-old Seymour to his parents from a summer camp in New England. It's a letter whose vocabulary and wisdom denote a godlike figure, with complex words, foreign phrases, and profound insights drooling like froth from its pages. This final story seemed to have no point except to show how otherworldly Seymour was as a boy. (Incidentally, in 1924, the date in the title of this story, Salinger himself was five years old.)

By this time, Seymour Glass had not only become an obsession, he had also become, perhaps, the final manifestation of the author's progressive narcissism and perhaps even paranoia—Seymour representing a projection of the author's own delusional belief that he himself was a Buddha-like figure in a world of phonies who were out to corrupt him.

Throughout his writings, Salinger was critical of psychotherapy, viewing therapists as part of the phony world, whose job it was to indoctrinate people. This view is common among narcissistic patients. The fact that Salinger was one of the most popular writers of his generation shows that many readers identified with his perspective, perhaps in part due to their own narcissistic features. By reading about the exalted Glass family, they could bask in its glory and also view themselves as pure souls in a corrupt world, thereby avoiding, just as Salinger had done, the reality of their own family conflicts and their own individual psychological problems. Thanks to Salinger's efforts, the defense mechanism of splitting—associated with borderlines and narcissists— reached an epidemic proportion: a whole generation assumed it was good and wise while splitting off and projecting its aggression onto others (the phonies).

A recent memoir, *Dream Catcher* (2000), by Salinger's daughter, Margaret, would seem to corroborate the view that the author underwent a psychological decline in his later years. She describes a father who was more tyrannical than Buddhist, who needed to control everyone around him, especially his wives and children. Among other things, she reported that he had an odd practice of drinking his own urine and administering a unique kind of acupuncture to his kids, using needles of his own device.

Salinger's "mirror" seems to have cracked. He didn't portray life objectively, but saw it through the prism of his psychopathology. Hence, while seeming to lead people toward a deeper insight, he was actually lighting the way toward a shared delusion. In his case, and in countless cases, emotional disturbances do not contribute to artistic success. How much greater would his output have been, and how much more objective and universal the content, had he not been sidetracked?

Artists are the spokespersons of their culture. From the time of the first cave paintings some 5,000 years ago, artists reflected what was going on in society—its mores, beliefs, and values. More than that, they have shown us at our best and at our worst, pointing out our triumphs and our defeats, our virtues and our vanities, our truths and our lies. They illuminate our deepest feelings, traveling where normal men and women fear to go. In a sense, they have a responsibility not only to themselves but also to society: a mission that requires that they and their "mirrors" are clear.

Chapter 2

Jessie and Joe:
Color and the Emotions

When she first entered treatment, there was something Jessie hated more than anything in the world. The problem arose when a friend commissioned her to do an oil painting. Jessie tried to convince the friend to accept one of her standard black-and-white sketches, but to no avail.

"I hate it!" she sighed. "I hate working with colors. I wish I didn't have to. I wish I had never been commissioned to do this painting." She had a whine in her voice, a forlorn expression in her eyes, a martyred stoop to her shoulders; yet the emotion she was displaying was somehow unconvincing. "I don't know why I can't just stick with black-and-white drawings. I like doing the drawings. I'm great at it. But deep inside I know I'll never respect myself as an artist unless I can master the use of color." She shook her head. "I really hate it."

She was a young artist who had come to therapy because, as she put it, she did not feel anything. Whenever I asked her during her once-a-week therapy sessions how she was feeling about her boss, her boyfriend, or about me, she would invariably reply that she felt nothing. She reported only numbness from her neck down. She thought feelings with her head but could not feel feelings with her body. As a result, she was not really connected to her art or to her life.

The plight of this patient was typical of many visual artists. Because she had gotten out of touch with her emotions, she had also lost touch with her creativity and her capacity to use colors. To the extent that artists repress their emotions, their use of color becomes limited or distorted—colors being visual representations of emotions. This repression happens unconsciously, without an artist knowing about it. On the surface they are aware only that they don't like working with color, and they often rationalize that color is not necessary or is not as artistic.

Usually this block about using color is connected to depression. In depression, all emotions—anger, fear, sadness, joy—are repressed. When repression reaches an extreme, as in this case, the person is left with a limited range of emotion. Feelings are frozen and replaced by an intellectual acknowledgement of feelings without actually sensing them in the peripheral nervous system. Along with this repression comes low self-esteem, a pessimistic outlook, and a lack of confidence. It is as if the repression of memories, and the emotions that are associated with them, jam up the brain, bringing about a general sense of ineptitude and futility. When a painter harbors a sense of ineptitude and futility, one of the first things that follows is a loss of confidence in using color.

Jessie first came to treatment following some disappointments in the New York art world. She could not get her drawings accepted into any galleries, not even the marginal ones in the East Village. Often, the galleries would ask if she had any oil paintings—implying that they wanted works that used color. She spent the first year of therapy talking about this issue, since she believed her salvation as a human being rested upon her success as an artist. Through fame, she would finally be worthy of her mother's love, since it was her mother who, as a failed artist herself, had pushed Jessie toward a career in art.

"What happens when you try to work in color?" I asked her again and again, hoping to enable her to understand her blocked feelings and how they were affecting her.

"I just . . . clamp up," she would say. She sat before me, her head nodding as usual, in a perfunctory way. "I don't have any confidence. I keep going over and over the faces, can't seem to get the noses right, or the mouths . . . and I can't do the shadows at all. It's ridiculous. When I paint in color I feel like a baby, as though I've never painted before. It's totally frustrating and humiliating."

"It's interesting that you say you feel like a baby. It makes me wonder what happened when you were a baby. It seems like you're stuck there." Gradually she remembered her childhood, and how she had formed the habit of numbing herself. When she was an infant several events combined to bring about this numbing. First, she was, according to her mother, a "difficult" baby who cried a lot. The physician recommended, according to the custom of that time, putting Valium (a tranquilizer) into her milk. This helped to soothe her, but it also made it doubly difficult for her to be weaned from the milk later on. Putting the

Valium in her milk created an addiction to using food not just for nutrition but also for self-soothing, which led to her having eating binges as an adult and weighing about seventy pounds more than she should have.

Second, she was weaned early because her mother had a succession of other children. Jessie found herself in the role of assistant mother, which meant she had to repress her own infantile needs and become an "adult" before she was developmentally ready.

A final factor in her development that affected her emotions was the physical abuse she suffered at the hands of both her mother and her father. Her parents were always fighting, and her father apparently displaced his anger with the mother onto the children. Jessie recalled that oftentimes she would hear them quarreling late at night, and then would be abruptly awakened. Her father would pick some reason to take it out on the kids. Perhaps they hadn't put away all their toys, or they had left the television set on when they went to sleep. He would wake them by whipping them with electrical wire (he was an electrician) while they were still in their beds. She learned to anticipate this by padding herself with extra clothing, but the events still left their emotional scars.

If Jessie yelled or cried, he would say, "Stuff it, or I'll give you something to really cry about." This process, over the years, helped to cement her habit of repressing her emotions. Indeed, individual colors were associated with particular feelings: the terror and rage associated with the beatings were connected with red, her loneliness with blue, and the tenderness that was missing in her infancy with yellow. In one sense, her inability to use those colors was an avoidance of the feelings and memories they would stir.

As the working-through process of therapy began to make inroads into these repressed emotions and memories, she reported flashes of anger, fantasies of revenge, and hints of sadness. This represented much progress for her, for until then she had experienced only anxiety—nothing else. However, she still could not effectively use color. Only when she could regularly have feelings in therapy did she acquire the capacity to do oil paintings in color. This took years of work, often utilizing a Gestalt approach. One such approach that worked well was the Paradoxical Exaggeration Technique.

"Are you feeling numb today?" I would ask.

"I suppose so. I don't feel anything, so I guess I must be numb."

"I'd like to try an experiment. I want you to make yourself even more numb."

"Why?"

"Maybe you're not numb enough to really block out all your feelings. Maybe you need to make yourself even number. Just trust me, and see what happens. I want you to deliberately concentrate on numbing yourself."

She sat up in her chair, shaking her head. "All right, if you say so." She stiffened herself, staring at me as she did so. "This feels funny."

"Funny?"

"Pins and needles."

"Do it even more."

"I don't know if I can."

"You can. You've been doing it all your life. You're a master at it."

"Yes, but not deliberately."

"Just do it."

She gritted her teeth. "It feels . . . "

"What?"

" . . . strange . . . " Suddenly she began to shake, then to sob. "What's happening to me?"

"Your sadness is coming up. The sadness you've been repressing. Keep going."

"I'm so scared."

"That's how you've felt all your life. That's how you felt back then."

She sobbed a few minutes, crying in brief stints, then stopping herself and catching her breath.

It took many sessions for her to allow herself to cry. First, she had to overcome the inhibition to crying that had been conditioned by her father's continually telling her, "Stuff it or I'll give you something to really cry about." Then we worked through the inhibition connected to her fear of losing control and of being vulnerable to more abuse. Finally, she regained her feelings, and her capacity for using color began to grow. She turned out oil paintings in muted colors, then oil paintings in brighter colors while, at the same time, she was becoming more optimistic and less depressed and self-disparaging. This, in turn, helped her to feel secure enough to maintain a long-term relationship with a man. Sometimes it takes a while for things to happen in therapy, and when they do, they sometimes snowball, as if automatically making up for lost time.

Joe was another artist I had worked with over the years who had difficulty with the use of color. He painted huge abstract canvases in fuzzy shades of black and gray. Indeed, there did not seem to be any order of any kind in the paintings; rather it was almost as if he had simply smeared his feces from corner to corner in some kind of frenzied fit. Like Jessie, he had trouble finding a gallery to show his work, and when he finally did convince an owner to at least include him in a group show, he didn't sell a single painting.

"All that work for nothing," he would moan in his sessions with me. "They really have no idea what my paintings are about."

"Why do you think that is?" I asked.

"Probably because the trend today is figurative art. Nobody wants abstract art anymore. They don't know what to make of it."

Every few months he would manage to get included in another group show. After each exhibition he would go through a post-show depression.

"Didn't sell a single painting," he would sigh, and then laugh sarcastically.

"Why do you think that is?" I would ask again.

"They just don't understand."

If I made even the slightest attempt at analyzing why his paintings were not appreciated, or let out even an inkling of a suggestion that perhaps they might be a bit bleak, he would glower and grunt with disdain.

"I'm not going to sell out. I don't care if nobody buys them. At least I have my integrity. Nobody can buy that."

His very sense of himself was somehow attached to his dark, messy paintings. If they had been dark and messy in some organized way, they might have been interesting. But they were dark and messy in a disorganized way and, as I said, had the look of black-on-black feces. You could almost smell them. I interpreted them as a kind of angry protest against the art world, which stood as a symbol of authority, which, on a deeper level, represented his parents, who had discouraged his artistic activity as a child and had in other ways enraged him. In other words, he was symbolically defecating on his parents.

In his paper on eroticism, Freud (1908a) described people who, as children, take a comparatively long time to overcome their infantile fecal incontinence. Such children go through a prolonged phase of anal eroticism, during which they will play with their feces and smear it on the objects around them, including the walls. As adults, such people tend to become stingy, orderly, and stubborn. They can also be anal-narcissistic, as I pointed out in a recent paper (Schoenewolf, 1996), and develop grandiose notions about themselves and their products. They will hold stubbornly to a position or point of view, even if it isn't working, because they are convinced, due to the grandiosity, that they and only they truly see things clearly.

Joe fit both Freud's description and mine. He was certainly stingy: He paid my minimum rate and did so grudgingly, complaining often that he couldn't afford it and that I wasn't helping him. He was orderly; this I knew because he told me he would sometimes clean and straighten his apartment several times a day. He was stubborn—most strikingly in the way he would "cut off his nose to spite his face" by refusing to change his style of painting even though he was tortured by the fact that his works weren't selling. Finally, he was grandiose, most notably with regard to his estimation of himself as an artist. Without having sold a single painting or having received any positive feedback about his work, he believed that he was a great artist whose paintings were simply too subtle and too original for people to understand. (Incidentally, there are cases in which a great artist's work *is* too original or subtle or daring to be appreciated—such as when Rodin's early erotic sculptures shocked Paris, prompting art critics and the public to call him a philistine—but this was not one of those cases.)

He also had a history in early childhood of anal incontinence. In Joe's case, his incontinence seemed to be connected, first, to his mother's depression. After his birth, she had two miscarriages, each of which left her in despair, so that she would lie in bed all day and not be able to administer to Joe's needs. Two years after Joe's birth, she finally had another child—a boy—at which time, she threw herself into the mothering of her new baby, assuaging her pent-up feelings through this activity. Hence, Joe went into the anal stage with only minimal supervision from his mother and, instead of things going smoothly, they went badly. He regressed and began to follow the example of his younger brother by remaining incontinent for a long time, and to angrily smear his feces on the wall next to his bed.

His father, a distant man who worked long hours and stayed away from home, added to Joe's discontent. What Joe usually remembered about his father was how he would promise things and then not deliver. One memory, for example, was of when his father had bought Joe a model airplane. They went out to fly it, and his father immediately wrecked it. "I'll get you another one next week," he said as they walked back to the car. He never did. Since his father never·delivered on his promises, Joe developed a pattern of not listening to his father's advice and of doing the opposite of what he advised. When it was time to pick a major in college, Joe chose art; his father had wanted him to become a doctor or a lawyer. Joe insisted on art, so his father reneged on his promise to pay for his college expenses. Joe stubbornly paid his own way, working at odd jobs while living in his car. He had the sense that this suffering somehow made him stronger.

When Joe finished college, his father wanted him to move back to his hometown, but Joe went to New York City to pursue a career as an artist. His art work during his first few years in the city was almost entirely a product of his neurosis. He struggled with each painting as if each were an act of constipated defecation. On a symbolic level, the paintings might have been seen as a reenactment of anal erotic soiling and smearing, as well as a defense against that smearing; hence, the internal conflict that caused the paintings to be "squeezed" out of him. In addition, each painting seemed to represent a symbolic act of "shitting" on his parents and on the art world. This wholesale shitting was a good example of what in behavioral psychology is called stimulus generalization. Nobody appreciated him, so everyone had to be shat on.

When I first interpreted these things for him, his reaction was disbelief. "That sounds like a bunch of psychoanalytic nonsense." I tried to point out how angry he was at his parents, citing the various memories he had disclosed during treatment. "Sure I'm angry at them. So what, everybody's angry at their parents."

"Well, where do you think that anger goes?"

"Where does it go? It doesn't go anywhere. It just stays inside me."

"It goes into your work. Your paintings are an angry protest. It's like you're saying to the world, 'Here. Take my anger. Eat it and love it.' And when the world doesn't particularly want your anger, you get even more angry."

"I like being angry," he replied. "That's what gives my art its edge. Of course my paintings are works of protest. What's wrong with that?"

Sometimes psychotherapy involves going over and over things like a record stuck in a groove. Joe and I must have had this same conversation a hundred or more times over several years. Gradually, very gradually, I was able to make some headway, particularly when I called attention to his father transference toward me. Just as he wouldn't listen to his own father, he wouldn't listen to me. He was convinced that, like his father, I wasn't supportive of his art career (even though my specialty is treating artists). Hence, when I made interpretations about his paintings being an angry protest against his parents, he viewed that as being unsupportive.

We began to focus more and more on his relationship with me. Soon he was saying, "*You* don't understand my work," just as he had once said, "*They* don't understand my work."

"What don't I understand?"

"You don't understand what I'm trying to do."

"Tell me about it. What are you trying to do?"

"If I have to explain it, forget it."

Whenever I asked that question, he would be evasive. It forced him to recognize that in fact he didn't have any idea of what he was trying to do. "I know exactly what I'm trying to do," he spat out. "But I don't really want to put it into words. Paintings aren't suppose to be explained. They are what they are. Either you get it or you don't."

Week after week the therapy focused on his paintings.

"In a way, you're just like my dad," he said one day. "You're always putting my work down."

"How do I put it down?"

"You're always telling me it's shit. That I'm shitting on the world. And you're always telling me to change my style and sell out."

"Are you saying you're not thinking of turds when you paint?"

"Sure, sometimes I'm thinking of turds. I think of a lot of things when I'm painting and sometimes, yes, I think of turds. What of it?"

"You may think of a lot of things, but the only thing I see in your paintings right now are dark black turds twisting this way and that. Maybe, if there were some green turds or pink turds, your paintings might be more interesting. Instead it's one painting after another of black turds."

"I happen to like black turds. So sue me."

"The point is, you're shitting on your audience, the very people whom you then resent for not buying your work. You're not using your talent properly; you're acting out of spite. You've come to me for advice and help, particularly with your art career. You've told me how much you struggle with each painting, how you don't really enjoy it, and how you torture yourself after each group show because you don't sell any of your paintings. My job is to try to help you understand why painting is such a struggle, how you can get to a point where it is more of a joy, and how you can support yourself, which is what you say you want. How can I do that without pointing out the psychodynamics that may be preventing you from achieving your aims?"

We had this same argument often during the course of several years. Finally one day, after yet another unsuccessful exhibition, he acknowledged that maybe, just maybe, his "turd paintings"—as he now called them—were ahead of the times. Maybe, just for the hell of it, he would try another variation.

A few weeks later he brought in a slide of a painting in which just a touch of red could be detected in one corner.

"Is that a red turd in the corner?" I asked.

He sort of sneered. "Yeah. I guess so."

A while later he showed me another slide with a trace of green. Still later came a slide with smidgens of yellow and blue. "Yeah, right. Two colors," he begrudgingly acknowledged.

The day he strode into the room with a grin on his face, I knew the "battle for color and spontaneity" had been won. "I finished a new painting today and I actually enjoyed doing it," he exclaimed before he had tumbled back onto my couch. "And you know what? It's gorgeous. It's really gorgeous! When Peggy saw it, she said, 'I hope you don't sell that painting, because I want it.' And there wasn't a single turd in it."

The painting was the first in which he used all of the primary colors, and it turned out to be the first of his paintings to sell.

Chapter 3

May: The Writer
Who Couldn't Be Serious

May was a successful writer when she started therapy. She was a frequent contributor of comedy skits to several popular television shows and was well-off financially. Many people would have envied her accomplishments. However, she was not at all satisfied with herself. First, she didn't really enjoy writing. She had to struggle all week to squeeze out two skits of three or four pages each, and she could only manage to do that after she had smoked a joint or two of marijuana. Second, her ambition was to be a serious writer, not a writer of witty skits, and this ambition had long been frustrated. Each time she tried to write something serious, it came out so melodramatic that it was unintentionally funny. She seemed "doomed" to write only commercial comedies.

"I'd like to write a novel about some of my darker experiences," she sighed during one of her first sessions with me. "But every time I sit down to write, I get restless, and I start thinking it's just going to be *schmaltzy* anyway, so why bother? Then before long I'm on the phone with a friend, wolfing down a box of marshmallow cookies. That's the story of my life."

She lay on my couch, an attractive, slightly plump woman in her thirties, fidgeting with the buttons of her blouse as she spoke. She was smiling, but only with her somewhat pouty mouth; in contrast, her sensitive blue eyes, magnified by her glasses, were like two beacons of anxiety blinking around the room.

"What's the story of your life?" I asked. "Restlessness or wolfing down a box of marshmallow cookies?"

"The whole thing. It's all such trite stuff. Very old. Like the plot of a detective novel."

"You know, you use that word a lot."

"What word?"

"Trite."

"Oh really? I didn't realize that."

The key to May's problem unfurled from that word. In Lacanian psychoanalysis, the word "trite" would be seen as a signifier, a clue to her unconscious process (Lacan, 1982). She couldn't empathize with herself. She saw herself as a trite heroine of a trite Gothic romance novel, whose problems were trite and whose childhood was even more trite. If she couldn't take herself seriously, how could she write a serious novel, in which she had to take seriously characters who were projections of herself? It was, as they say, a conundrum.

May was the youngest child and only daughter of a wealthy couple from Long Island, raised in a large, Gothic house near the bay, where the mornings were misty and the evenings were dark and mysterious. She had a brother who was eight years older, who seemed more like a crazy uncle than a brother. On the surface, her story did have the appearance of a cliché: the typical story of a poor little rich girl who had had many material advantages but whose spirit had been squashed. However, under the surface her life was anything but a cliché.

Shengold (1979) used the term "soul murder" (borrowing it from an autobiography of schizophrenic Daniel Paul Schreber, about whom Freud wrote a case history) to describe the kind of child rearing in which "the victim is robbed of his identity and of the ability to maintain authentic feelings" (p. 557). He believed that certain very disturbed caretakers did this by sexually, physically, and emotionally abusing a child while at the same time acting as if all was normal. When children are abused and told the abuse is normal, they don't learn to empathize with themselves or to know what is real, and this is devastating to their development.

In May's case, her mother seems to have suffered from some kind of severe disorder. It could have been schizophrenia or multiple personality disorder. Here are some of May's memories of her mother: When she was about three years old, her mother caught May fingering her clitoris. Her mother punished her by putting ice cubes in May's panties. When she was four and five her mother would masturbate in front of her in the bathtub. She recalled occasions, when she was six or seven, during which her mother would coo sweetly about how much she loved her and seconds later would be chasing her around the kitchen table with a bread knife. She recalled never being able to bring a friend home without her mother doing something bizarre to scare the friend away. Her childhood was quite isolated.

As May grew up, her mother carefully arranged her entire life. Her mother picked her clothing until the day she graduated from college. She signed her up for piano lessons, figure-skating lessons, horseback-riding lessons, tennis lessons, painting lessons, violin lessons, skiing lessons, ballet lessons, and every other kind of lesson she thought a refined young lady should have. May's whole life was carefully controlled and monitored and there was not a second for her to stop and think about anything. If May uttered a word of complaint, her mother would become enraged and give her a long lecture about how lucky she was to have been born in such a well-to-do family and to be so privileged as to do all these things.

In the meantime, May's older brother enlisted her from a very early age as his "lover," while her mother looked the other way. May recalled being awakened by him almost every morning, beginning at about the age of three or four, at which time he would fondle her and have her perform oral sex on him. As she grew older, he began to start the days by having intercourse with her, referring to her as his "special sister-wife." On Saturday afternoons they would often go snake hunting, venturing out to a field near their house to find garter snakes under rocks. At some point he would ask her to find *his* snake, and she would dutifully unzip his fly and perform oral sex.

Her father, a banker and entrepreneur, was away from home much of the time. When he was home, May would run up to him and try to tell him what was happening to her. He would pick her up and hug her and call her "Daddy's girl," but he didn't believe anything she reported about her brother and her mother. He said she had a vivid imagination and encouraged her to become a writer. This meager encouragement from her father was all she needed. Her imagination soared.

While she rushed from painting to figure-skating to dance lessons, she would make up stories in her head about princesses who were rescued by princes from the hands of evil stepmothers. But she dared not write these stories down out of a fear that her mother might find them and be angry at her, or even worse, sign her up for writing lessons.

During her college days, she began to experiment with drugs and sex. Fortunately, she was intelligent enough that she could make As and Bs while seldom attending classes. If she couldn't pass the exams, she would sleep with the professor. By the time she graduated, she was using cocaine almost daily and working as a call girl. Her father, who had since died, had set up a trust fund for her, but her mother had appropriated it and spent all the money on cruises around the world. May ended up having to pay for her final year of college by signing up with various escort agencies.

"It was easy for me to have sex with guys for money because I wasn't really 'there,'" she explained. "My body was there, but it was like a mannequin—devoid of feelings or even the twitch of a nerve-ending. Not only was I constantly stoned, but also I had no self, no identity. I had been programmed by my mother to be this Barbie doll extraordinaire, and I had grown quite good at acting the part. I'd also become an expert at submitting myself sexually, since I'd been doing that for my brother all my childhood, but, as I said, I wasn't really there; I was in my head, looking at the whole thing and thinking about how someday I'd write about it. Night after night I'd go out with these sleazy older guys, and I'd be oh so clever and coy, and they'd love the hell out of me, and I'd sniff some more cocaine, and all the while I hadn't a clue who I was. Not a clue."

It was at this time that she was resourceful enough to get herself an agent and had him submit some of her comedy skits to a famous television comedy show. They were accepted, and soon she became a regular contributor to this and other comedy shows. She managed to eke out two or three of these skits a week between escort assignments and cocaine parties. But somehow, through it all, she knew that something important was missing—something quite essential to an authentic life—her real self.

"I tried to write a story last week," she would sigh during her sessions.

"How'd it go?"

"The same. I couldn't finish it. It was stupid."

"Why do you think it was stupid?"

"Because it was. Whenever I try to write a serious story, especially if it's autobiographical, it turns out stupid."

"What do you mean by stupid?"

"Trite. Maudlin. Insipid. I don't know how to write about myself, since I don't have any idea of who I am. And so I write these trite stories about this trite Barbie doll character who lives a trite, maudlin Manhattan life, feeling sorry for herself because she was given all the material things but no love, blah, blah, blah."

"What do you think is really going on?"

"I don't know. I just feel this emptiness inside. This eternal, relentless emptiness. I can't talk about it."

This is how May's therapy sessions went for a long while. Even though she had had a very traumatic childhood, it was hard for her to write about or talk about herself. This is true of many patients in the beginning of therapy. She had not separated, emotionally, from her parents; hence, she still saw herself, unconsciously, through their eyes. Whenever she had complained about anything to her mother, her mother had reminded her of how "spoiled rotten" she was and how much was being given to her. Whenever she had complained about anything to her father, he would pat her head and tell her things were not really that bad. Now, as a young woman, it was still difficult for her to talk about herself, for there was always an inner voice (her mother's, her father's) telling her not to complain.

In psychoanalytic terms, she had an almost nonexistent ego. Hence, her superego, which embodied her mother's expectation that she be Barbie extraordinaire, was in a constant conflict with her id, which rebelled against her mother's expectations through escape into drugs and sex. There was no ego to mediate between the two—no integrated self, only these raging extremes of personality.

Fortunately, she did have her talent, which in a way became her salvation, as it does for many people in the arts. Her capacity to write funny skits and to make a good living from them, so that she could eventually stop working as a call girl, gave her something to be proud of and something on which to build an ego. In May's case, one could clearly see how nature and nurture (or lack of nurture) had combined to produce mixed results. She had inherited beauty and intelligence and talent, but those characteristics had been marred by the trauma of her upbringing and/or a genetic predisposition toward the kind of borderline impulsivity that was so prominent in her mother's life, as well as in her older brother's.

Comedy skits with a satirical, slightly macabre slant to them were easy for her to write. Freud noted in "Jokes and Their Relation to the Unconscious" (1905) how humor is used to express disguised aggression "in order to make aggressiveness or criticism possible against persons in exalted positions who claim to exercise authority. The joke then represents a rebellion against that authority, a liberation from its pressure" (p. 105). May's comedy skits were largely vehicles in which her anger at her family could be sublimated through artistic displacement: instead of making fun of her family, she could make fun of authority figures such as prominent politicians, portraying them as dictatorial, perverse, and misguided buffoons. However, although writing these skits provided her with some immediate gratification, it could not resolve the underlying complexity of feelings and memories. Without this resolution, her range of emotions and of writing styles remained narrow.

Artists require a special kind of therapeutic approach. First, you must demonstrate an understanding of the importance of the arts, either by showing that you yourself are an artist or that you have the sensitivity to appreciate art. This helps create a good working alliance. Second, you must understand that artists have a special sensitivity, which makes them susceptible to emotional disorders. Third, you must understand that artists must be artists and can't be fulfilled unless they actualize their creativity in some way.

The first hurdle in May's therapy was to assist her in taking herself seriously so that she could properly actualize her gifts. This meant helping her to work through her resistance to remembering and then her resistance to talking about how her writer's block related to traumatic aspects of her childhood.

"Do I really have to talk about all that?" she would ask, grimacing and sighing, looking back at me. "It's too depressing. I've spent years trying to forget it, and now you want me to remember it?"

"That's right, you've spent years running away from the depression inside you. And what did it get you? You've had to stay stoned on drugs the whole time."

"But if I start remembering things, I'm afraid I'll—I don't know what."

"Go crazy?"

"Maybe. Or I'll sink into a major depression."

"Believe me, you won't. Actually, you're in a depression now, but you've been hiding it from yourself. By remembering the traumas and talking about them and letting them out of your system, the depression will gradually go away. Also, it's important for you to tell them to somebody—to me; it's a way of reestablishing trust with the world."

She had to talk about the traumas, whether she wanted to or not. Like a woman in labor, her time had come; her repression had started to break. She talked in bits and pieces, halting her way through the maze, excavating a feeling here and a memory there. When it got too intense for her, she would call and cancel a session, but the next week she would come back with an anxious expression on her face, bearing new feelings and new memories. Sometimes this new material had been aroused by an event in her present life.

"Guess what my mother sent me? She sent me one of her care packages. Every now and then she sends these stupid care packages filled with hand-me-downs, and I received one today, out of the blue. Guess what was wrapped up in the clothes. Knives."

"Knives? What kind of knives?"

"Kitchen knives. Big, kitchen knives. They were wrapped up in some old second-hand dresses of hers. She always sends me her second-hand clothes, and I immediately give them away to homeless people on my block. She's done it since I was a teenager, because we wear the same size. I keep telling her they're not my style and not to send them, but she sends them anyway. This time there were all these knives wrapped in them. Used kitchen knives—you know, like a butcher knife and bread knife and such. It really terrified me."

"How come?"

"They were just like the knives she used to have in her kitchen. And when I saw them, I suddenly had a memory." She paused, hugging herself, glancing about with her anxious, bulging eyes as if she expected her mother to trounce through the door at any moment.

"Yes. What was it?"

"I remembered how she used to chase me with one of those knives in her hand. She would laugh like a witch. She would actually cackle. I'm serious. I was so terrified. She thought it was a big joke." She sobbed for a while, and then became thoughtful. "Why do you think she sent me those knives?"

"Why do *you* think?"

"It's almost as if she wanted to remind me of them, to keep me in the clutches of terror."

"Perhaps. At any rate, that's how you feel."

"Do you think I should call her and tell her how I feel about the knives, or ignore it?"

"What would happen if you called her and told her how you felt?"

"She'd immediately throw it back to me and ask me how I could say such a thing to her. She'd tell me I was being paranoid again. That's what she always told me as a child when I mentioned anything about what she or my brother were doing."

"Sounds like it wouldn't be fruitful to call her."

"No. Not at all. I should just talk about it in therapy, right?"

On another occasion, she received a telephone call from her brother (with whom she hadn't spoken in years). He wanted to know if she still had the violin, which she had learned, grudgingly, to play as a child. He wanted to present it to his daughter as a birthday present. When May replied that she had given it away to a homeless man, he was appalled. That same day her mother called her to lecture her about giving the violin away. "How could you be so thoughtless? Didn't it occur to you that your niece might need it someday?"

"This is how it always was," May observed in the following session. "The two of them were always teaming up against me. Maybe I should just cut off my relationships with both of them."

"Perhaps, until you find a way to relate to them without getting hurt."

As we proceeded with the working-through process, May's ego became stronger and stronger. Along with ego strength came higher self-esteem, more of a capacity to tolerate sadness, and a deepening ability to empathize with herself. While this was happening, she all at once stopped taking drugs and instead began stuffing herself with an array of vitamins and minerals. (She may have been going overboard in this respect—as some people tend to do—in an attempt to find a replacement for her oral-gratification needs, but it was certainly better than taking drugs.) I also noted that she made fewer and fewer self-depreciatory jokes about herself and that she could recall and talk about the sad times she had gone through and not blame herself for them. The squeamish look she often wore as she lay on the couch in the shadows of the afternoons was transformed into one of curiosity.

She had been in therapy for about a year and a half when she started working on a novel. "I don't quite understand it. The words seem to be oozing out of me. Maybe it's just a mirage. Maybe tomorrow I'll be blocked again. Oh, God, I hope not. Do you think it's just a mirage, Dr. S? Please say it's not."

"It's not," I said. "What's the novel about?"

"Can't talk about it while the flavor lasts."

The novel became a part of the therapy. Every week she came in full of new vitality, bearing new memories that had been aroused, in part, by the novel (which, I gleaned, was autobiographical). She would spend part of each session chattering excitedly about how well the novel was going—and it was reparative for her to be able to do that and get an encouraging response from me—and then relate the new memories that had come up and cry about them. It appeared that the strengthening of her ego by the act of writing helped to give her the sense of stability she needed in order to allow herself to recall the traumas and let them go.

Several months later she reported, "I showed part of the novel to my agent. He loved it. He took it right to this publisher he knows and they offered me a contract based the first few chapters. Can you believe it?"

"Congratulations."

She kept talking about her memories in therapy and writing the novel. Eventually she needed to talk about the memories less and enjoyed her writing more. The childhood wounds were healing, and she was able, not without effort, to forgive her family and resume a distant, guarded relationship with them. She began to see them not as powerful victimizers, but as fragile beings whose sense of well-being she could have destroyed with a few sentences of truth. Not destroying them when she knew that she could have, letting them hold on to their delusions, gave her a quiet confidence in her dealings with them and a growing sense of ego integrity and self esteem.

May went on to become a successful novelist and to also find fulfillment in other aspects of her life. That's how it usually works; the creative block is associated with an overall impingement that has an effect on both professional and personal provinces. When the block is dissolved, life moves on in all its splendor and misery.

Chapter 4

Leo:
The Actor Who Couldn't Cry

"I've never remembered a single dream, and as far as I know, I don't dream," he said resolutely. A handsome man in his early thirties, with a body that was tanned and muscled, he sat alertly before me, ready to plunge into therapy as he had plunged into other projects in his life. "I've spent my young adulthood working day and night, making large sums of money, devoting myself totally to my work while neglecting my social life. I'm your typical workaholic. I've dated men and women, but I never really feel anything emotionally for the people I date. After a while, they become too demanding, and I have to back off. All this has become boring to me of late. During the past year, I've started to wonder where my life is heading, so I sold my businesses and took a year off to study acting and find myself. However, I'm having a little problem in my acting classes. I can't cry. I don't know how important that is. I suppose I should be able to cry if I want to be a serious actor. That's what brought me here. I don't know if I'll be able to bring in any dreams, though. Does everybody dream?"

This "announcement" had come on the heels of my having explained, during our first session, that my method of therapy included the interpretation of dreams. "Yes," I told him. "Everybody dreams. But some people don't remember them. It takes practice."

He seemed skeptical. "Are you sure everybody dreams? I really don't think I do."

"Trust me. You do."

"Then why don't I remember them?"

"Probably for the same reason you can't cry."

Leo was a guy who believed he could solve any problem through hard work and determination. If you gave him a business problem, he could figure it out it in a minute. He had tried to apply this problem-solving method to his life and to the pursuit of his acting career, and it hadn't worked, so he had come to me in the hope that I could help him fine-tune his problem-solving approach.

He sat back in his chair and gazed at me intently, as if he were conducting an interview with a business client. "So, what do you think I can do to learn to cry as an actor? Are there some techniques you could recommend?"

"What happens when you have a scene that requires you to cry?"

"Nothing. I don't feel anything."

"Have you tried doing emotional recalls?" I asked, referring to a technique in Stanislavski's method of acting in which an actor recalls an incident in his past when he cried and uses that in the present role.

"Yeah, but I can't remember ever crying."

"You never cried as a kid?"

"I don't remember my childhood."

"Just like you don't remember dreams."

"Right. Do you think that's important? To remember dreams?"

"I think it could be very helpful in your case. I think if you could remember dreams, you could cry."

"Let's do it then!"

Freud often compared psychoanalytic therapy to an archeological dig, wherein the therapist and patient dig around in the patient's unconscious, uncovering bits and pieces of "ancient ruins." One of the ways of doing that is through a form of mental excavation called dream interpretation. In Leo's case I knew that his inability to remember dreams was connected to his being out of touch with his feelings. Hence, I decided that his dreams would be the avenue through which we could get him reconnected. However, it took several months before he was able to bring in his first dream. It and many that followed were about his three cats.

In the first dream, a good friend picked up one of his cats and was trying to throw it out the window. At the last minute, Leo grabbed the cat from the friend's hands. In another, a rat crawled into the anus of one of his cats, causing the cat to screech in pain. (This image is similar to one dreamed by Freud's famous patient, "the Rat Man.") In another, he came home to find one of his cats with a gaping wound on its head. The cat died in agony as he looked on helplessly. In yet another, all three of Leo's cats had mysteriously disappeared while he was out shopping.

"It seems that in all these dreams, bad things are happening to your cats," I said to him. "What do you make of that?"

"I guess I'm afraid, really terrified, that something bad will happen to them."

"Why are you so concerned about them?"

"I'm not sure."

"How do you feel about your cats?"

"They're more important to me than anything else in my life, certainly more than any people. I love my cats. If anything happened to them, I don't know what I'd do. They're the loves of my life."

He was not a beastialist, per se; he didn't make love to his cats. But in a broader sense, he had libidinalized them—investing them with more of his emotions than any of the humans in his life. When he wanted love and comfort, he went to them. In the middle of the night when he couldn't sleep, he drew them around his sides, held them tightly, and whispered "sweet nothings" to them. "Yes, yes, yes, I love you!" he would utter. The threat of losing them aroused in him the kind of separation anxiety most people feel with regard to their loved ones.

"What thoughts come to your mind when you think of something bad happening to your cats?" I asked him one day.

"I just remembered something," he said, his eyes lighting up with surprise at this strange act of remembering, which heretofore had been so alien to him. "When I was very small, I had this big stuffed cat, and I used to sleep with it and take it everywhere. My mother kept telling me that it was getting old and that I should throw it away, but I didn't want to. If she tried to take it away from me, I'd cry and cry. Once she put it on top of the refrigerator where I could see it but not touch it. Then she relented and gave it back. Then one day it disappeared for good. I don't remember asking her about it. I knew she had thrown it away, and I guess I didn't feel I could say anything to her about it."

"How come you couldn't say anything to her?"

"You just couldn't. If she decided to do something, that was that. Case dismissed, you know? Actually, that brings another memory to mind. Later on, I used to get attached to certain T-shirts, and again she'd nag me about throwing them away, and then one day I'd find them missing in action. I never said anything about the missing T-shirts either.

"Wow, I just thought of another memory. I don't know if this is connected or not. But I just remembered that my parents didn't want me to play with the neighborhood kids. It was like they were beneath me in some way, and I might get contaminated or something. My mother would have the same expression when she talked about these kids as when she talked about my old T-shirts. Yeah, it seems that they never allowed me to get attached to anything or anyone. Right! Later on in high school, both my parents were always critical of the people I hung out with, like they were frivolous, not serious-minded enough. When I had my first girlfriend—during my senior year—and they caught us having sex in my room, they demanded that I break up with her immediately. They acted like she was some slut who was trying to distract me from my mission. " 'You should be concentrating on your studies, preparing for college,' they kept telling me. I mean, I could understand their getting a little upset, but they really got ticked off and wouldn't let it drop for months. They still bring it up today, as if it were some kind of major betrayal."

Now, at the age of thirty-three, it had dawned on him that he had never taken a vacation, nor even permitted himself a day or two of relaxation; that is, he had never really taken time for his personal life. He had come to realize that he had been, as he put it, "on automatic pilot." This had prompted him to give up his businesses and come to New York to pursue what for his parents was the most frivolous notion of all—acting. They had tried frantically to talk him out of it, but this time, for the first time, he had refused to listen to them.

He had thrown himself into acting as he did everything else, but he soon realized he was self-conscious about playing the roles assigned to him and unable to be genuine as he intoned his lines. This took him by surprise; he had thought that he would be able to translate his business acumen and his ability to project a confident air to the art of acting, even when he didn't feel confident. But as an actor, he was required to show his real self through his roles, something he hadn't needed to do as a businessman. Indeed, he had an extreme fear, almost a terror, of public exposure. In this sense, acting was for him a counterphobic activity and the journey to New York was an attempt at self-therapy. He had been taught that his real feelings were indulgences, and he was also afraid of being exposed as a fraud. This sense of being a fraud, we soon discovered, was linked with an inflated self-image and an underlying guilt, which we traced to factors in his childhood.

Leo was the only male child—"the golden boy"—of his family. Although he had a twin sister, he was always given preferential treatment by both his mother and his father. Leo came from a patrilineal family and was made aware from an early age that, as the son, he would be carrying on the family name. His father, who had achieved some success in business, wanted his son to follow in his footsteps and take the family name to a higher level. His mother conveyed to him that he was a special person who could do anything that he set his mind to.

This preferential treatment became even more obvious when a sister was born. Often a younger sibling replaces the older sibling in the mother's eyes, and the mother dotes on the baby. In this case, the baby sister was almost totally ignored by both parents, while they continued to tout their golden boy. This sister developed an eating disorder, grew obese, and the mother continually nagged her about her weight, an attitude which only served to keep the girl overweight. Ironically, during latency, Leo also became overweight, but the parents said nothing to him about it.

Throughout his childhood, Leo saw but could not acknowledge to himself that he was the golden boy who received preferential treatment over his sisters. Unconsciously, however, he felt a great deal of guilt about this situation, and it affected his developing self-image. "I felt rotten inside, as though I were in some way contributing to the mistreatment of my sisters by going along with my parents." Leo felt good when his mother and father always praised him, putting him on a pedestal, but the side effect was a wedge between him and his sisters. Grave doubts were aroused about whether he deserved so much attention, and he put constant pressure on himself to live up to their expectations of him. He also discovered there were other strings attached to the devotion of his parents. They required that he in turn be attached to nothing else and nobody else but them (hence, the removal of the objects and people in his life to which he became attached); they required that he live out their own ambitions (become a superachiever); and they required that he idealize them and overlook any of their faults.

One memory underscored this last requirement. One summer day when Leo was about eight, his mother gave a party, for which she made some pizza. Upon taking a bite of the pizza, Leo exclaimed, "Mom, you made this pizza too spicy." His mother purportedly lost her temper. "What do you mean, 'too spicy'? Who do you think you are, young man—a prince? What the hell do you know about spice, anyway? This pizza is just fine, and I don't want to hear another word about it."

He described his mother as being overly affectionate—smothering him with it—but with a tendency, as illustrated above, to turn on him if he didn't mirror her exactly as she wanted him to. On the other hand, his father was cold and distant. Leo remembered a situation that seemed to epitomize his father's relationship with him. When Leo was about six years old, he stole some small objects from a toy store and when his father found out about it, he drove the boy back to the store and had him give them back to the clerk and admit that he had stolen them. Then his father drove Leo back home and sat sternly on a chair in Leo's bedroom as the boy lay in bed crying. He recalled feeling angry, lonely, guilty, and confused about everything. At one point he looked up, wanting to explain why he had done it and how he had been feeling. "Dad?" he called out. He got no reply. "Dad?" he said again. His father stared at him with his stern, unforgiving eyes and said, "Are you finished crying?" Leo nodded that he was. "Good!" his father said and strode out of the room. That's the last time Leo ever remembered crying.

There was never any attempt by the father to find out what Leo was feeling. His father never cried, never complained, and was always stoic about everything. He expected the same of his son. Their relationship was like that of a drill instructor and his recruit, the father always quietly but firmly pressing him to achieve. If Leo did what was expected, he received a silent, grudging smile of approval. If he didn't, he was met with a cold stare.

In college, Leo divided his time between his studies and his businesses. He ran several business operations during those years, enabling him not only to completely pay for his college but also to put money into stocks and bonds. After college he expanded one of the businesses and started two new ones. By the time he had reached his mid-twenties, he had several employees working for him. He was always on the go and managed only about five hours of sleep each night.

Meanwhile, his personal life remained somewhat of a confusing nuisance to him. Being handsome and industrious, people of both sexes were attracted to him, and he slept with whoever offered himself or herself to him. However, he kept his distance from both men and women. He experienced any rejection by either a woman or a man as a narcissistic injury. Such rejections would catapult him into a depression in which he was deluged by feelings of guilt, anger, and confusion (perhaps the same feelings that overwhelmed him as he had lain in his room crying, his father watching him sternly). To avoid these feelings at all costs, he would try to make sure he was always in control. He would never pursue anybody, but would wait for people to come to him. "I'm always on top of the situation, always the one who's admired," he explained. "For a while I get off on that. But before long it gets boring, and they become too demanding of my time, so I have to end it." He would get rid of ex-lovers the same way he fired people in his businesses.

With women he was interested only in sex and was disgusted by any show of tenderness, afraid that it was going to turn into the kind of smothering love he had received from his mother. Eventually he would come to see them as fallen women. "Any woman who sleeps with me has to be a whore," he noted one day and then had an association: "Of course, that's how my parents felt about the first girl I had sex with in high school." With men, he was less interested in sex than in their physical affection. "I always craved affection from my dad," he speculated. "Perhaps I'm displacing my frustration? I know it's more important to me to be hugged by a man than to have sex with him. I have sex with men sort of out of obligation."

In the end, he would withdraw from the "complications" of relationships with humans and draw comfort from his cats. Night after night he found himself alone with them. It was he and the cats against the world. He treated them with the care and understanding that he wished he had had as a boy, feeding them food from his own table, buying them the best toys, dressing them in the finest collars. If one purred a little loudly during the night, he would immediately take it to a veterinarian. They were always in his lap, and he constantly sang to them and nurtured them. Before going to sleep each night, he would give each about ten kisses.

"They're the only things that matter to me," he said once, and he appeared to be on the verge of tears, but stopped himself. "That's sad, isn't it? Isn't that sad?"

In analyzing his relationship with his cats, I thought of Winnicott's (1965) emphasis of the role of transitional objects in childhood development. He explained that a transitional object such as a doll, teddy bear, blanket, piece of cloth, or old shoe—or a transitional phenomena such as thumb-sucking or masturbation—serves to help a child make the transition from his own "subjective reality" to "shared reality" with another person and constituted a form of self-soothing. The problem is that the object, which is generally first embraced by the child at about ten months of age and held onto for several years, generally becomes smelly and filthy, and most mothers can't help becoming disgusted.

However, taking away this transitional object can be harmful to the child's development.

To illuminate this point, Winnicott asks, How can normal children lose their homes and all that is familiar to them and not become ill? The answer, of course, is that they have their transitional objects to soothe the transition. This is the first object the child can really call his or her own, and which is always there for the child:

> If we deprive a child of the transitional objects and disturb the established transitional phenomena, then the child has only one way out, which is a split in the personality, with one half related to a subjective world and the other reacting on a compliance basis to the world which impinges. (1965, p. 144)

Winnicott goes on to assert that when this split is formed and the child can't integrate the subjective and the objective, the child is "unable to operate as a total human being" (p. 145). He concludes, in typical Winnicottian language:

> the world is never as we would create it and . . . the best that can happen for any one of us is that there shall have been sufficient overlap of external reality and what we can create. We accept the idea of an identity between the two as an illusion. (p. 144)

His rather pessimistic view of the possibility of merging internal and external reality notwithstanding, his notions about transitional objects seem applicable to Leo's case. His first transitional object, the stuffed cat, was taken away from him when he was about two or three years old. He had needed this object to help him adjust to the demands of reality and as a means of self-soothing. When this object was taken away from him, he began to split himself into two parts, the conscious part—the golden boy, the dutiful son, the superachiever—and the unconscious part—his real feelings, which he learned to hide from himself.

In a sense he was stuck at an early stage of emotional development, fixated at the point at which he was deprived of his transitional object. Subsequent events in his childhood had reinforced this fixation—his being isolated from his sisters and from playmates, his being driven to achieve, his being discouraged from crying or any emotionality. The cats in his present life were replacements for the original transitional object, and they still served the same function of the original stuffed cat;

they were intended to be a bridge to help him adapt to reality and to soothe him. Unfortunately, while the cats could offer him a limited comfort, they couldn't help him to learn to relate to humans or to figure out how to be real as an actor. Only therapy could help him do that.

Now and again he would bring in more dreams about his cats. The riddle of these dreams that continued to elude him was: Why was something bad always happening to his cats? In the beginning, I held back on answering that question, not wanting to tell him something he was not yet ready to hear. He had been in treatment for seven or eight months before I made the first interpretation.

"You know those cats you always dream about?" I asked one day.

"Yes. *My* cats. What about them?"

"Well, have you ever wondered why you keep making them sick and torturing them and killing them off?"

"I don't kill them. Other people kill them."

"But you dreamed the dreams. You made up the plots in which bad things are done to your cats."

"I don't know if I buy that."

It took him several months to take in and digest that thought, during which time I repeated it again and again. Only after he had completely accepted it did I go to the next step.

"I wonder whether the cats in your dreams could also represent yourself. In other words, when you pet and soothe your cats, it's almost as if you were soothing yourself—that is, soothing your inner child as symbolized by the cats."

"I can see that. That rings true."

"In that case, perhaps we can finally solve the riddle of why you keep having bad things happen to your cats in your dreams."

"Oh, yeah?"

"If the cats are you, then perhaps having bad things happen to them is a way of punishing yourself (in symbolic form) to assuage your guilt feelings."

"I don't follow you."

"You keep talking about how guilty you feel about leading people on and rejecting them. And you've talked about how guilty you feel about the double standard your parents applied to you and to your two sisters—how they treated you like a prince and them like paupers. And you've talked about how whenever you act, you're always afraid you're going to be exposed as a fraud. When I've asked you what you meant by 'fraud,' you've always associated it with your guilt feelings.

"For instance, two of your dreams were about a man with whom you went out for a short time and then rejected because, as you put it, he became too demanding of your time. In your dreams, you have him trying to throw your cats out of the window and you have a rat crawling into the anus of one of your cats (symbolic perhaps of this man anally penetrating you). These dreams may represent your guilt feelings about this man."

"I never thought of that. It could be."

It was not until much later, after he had been in therapy for a year and a half, that I gave him the final interpretation of the dream.

"Many times in dreams, situations are reversed," I told him after he had brought in yet another cat dream. "For example, in your dreams about cats, you have bad things happen to your cats, often done by others. People seem to be angry at your cats and to want to hurt them. We've talked about the guilt factor, but there's also an anger factor. These people seem to be angry at your cats (at you). Why do you suppose they're so angry?"

"Because I've rejected them, usually."

"Right. In other words, the anger in the dream is really your own anger in reverse. You harbor unconscious anger toward the people around you, but in the dreams you have them angry at your cats."

"I'm not aware of feeling angry at anybody. I just feel impatient with them."

"What do you think of when you think of angry people?"

"Losers. Getting angry means you've lost. That's how my father always made me feel."

This one took a while to sink in. It's easy for people to look at what other people are doing to them. Most people first come into therapy because they want a supportive ear with regard to how they are being deprived or abused by the world. However, getting people to look at themselves objectively, and to consider what they may be doing to others, how they may be unwittingly acting out anger, or how they may be deluding themselves, is another matter. Confucius once said, "I have looked far and wide and have not been able to find a man who could bring home the judgment against himself."

I knew that Leo was in a rage at his parents because they had made him into a narcissistic extension of themselves. They were "stage parents" and he the dutiful son who would achieve for them. Meanwhile, he was conditioned not to have a personal life and not to have feelings and to treat others the same way his parents had treated him. He had admired his father and basked in his father's light, but ultimately felt deprived by him. Now people admired him and he allowed them, for a time, to bask in his own light before he gave them the "cold shoulder," as he put it. I knew this interconnected fabric of unconscious conflicts lay at the root of his actor's block. The problem was he couldn't allow himself to look objectively at his parents, which he needed to do in order to make the transition from transitional object to human object. And in order for him to look objectively at his parents, he first had to look objectively at himself.

His primary concern, of course, was about his acting. Most of his sessions were spent talking about what was happening in his acting classes. Since that was where his primary focus lay, that was where I also focused my attention. However, in focusing on acting, we had to talk about his feelings—or lack thereof—and about his associations. Invariably these associations led to what was going on in his life, and what had gone on in his past. This gave me the opportunity to bring to his attention how he was stuck in a mode of operation in which he was blocking his emotions generally and acting them out—particularly anger and guilt. Eventually he did admit to being angry.

The first conscious target of his anger was myself; he wanted to "kill the messenger" for pointing out this anger to him. He felt I was criticizing him just as his father had done, and he developed an intense, negative father transference toward me. He went through a period in which he missed sessions or came in and was belligerent, and during which he frequently threatened to quit therapy. One day, for example, he brought his bicycle into my waiting room and sat it there. When I asked him how I should feel about that, he snarled. "Actually, I don't really care. I came in thinking I would quit therapy today anyway."

It was in the middle of this period that Leo first cried. He had come in angrily as usual, sat upright on the couch, refusing to lie down, and threatened to quit therapy for the umpteenth time.

"Why should I keep coming here? Nothing's happening. It's not helping. All that's happening is that I'm getting more depressed and angry. Why continue?"

"You're right; we seem to be stuck. I have an idea. How about if we do an acting exercise?" I suggested.

"What kind of exercise?"

"Let's do a scene. Let's say I'm a teacher, very much like myself, and you're a student, very much like yourself. And you're angry at this teacher for reasons very similar to the ones that make you angry at me. Okay? Now this scene is the day in which you finally give it to me. The big tell-off scene, where you tell me everything you think of me and were too polite to say."

He looked at me incredulously, but with a glint of anticipation. "You want me to tell you off."

"That's right."

He was silent for a moment, then leaped up from the couch. "Fine. Is it all right if I walk around?"

"All right. But no hitting. I have this aversion to being slugged." I was being serious and silly at the same time, trying to goad him a bit.

"Right. Right. Okay." He began pacing the floor. I could see him working himself up to it. Finally he started. "You know. There's something I've been meaning to tell you. I really hate your guts." He stopped as if surprised at himself. "Actually, I really do hate your guts. I don't know why. But I do, and actually, this isn't part of the scene anymore. I really do hate your guts, and it feels good to say it." He glared at me, smiling with delight. "In fact, fuck you. That's my tell-off speech to you. Fuck you. Fuck you in the ass! How do you like that?" He cackled nervously and continued. "You think you know everything, don't you? I'm just supposed to come here and listen to you like you're some kind of god and I'm a devout worshipper. I'm supposed to come here and spill out my guts and meanwhile you sit there and you don't say shit about how you're feeling or what your thinking. You're holding everything back, and I'm the big sucker who's sitting here spilling my guts and you sit there and criticize me. Fuck that. And fuck you. And if you don't like my saying that, fuck you again! Why don't you say something? Don't know what to say, do you?"

He went on like this for a while, and as I observed him, I found myself feeling sad. I understood that on the transferential level he wasn't talking about me at all, but about his father. However, this was not the time for an interpretation. When he had finished his tirade, he suddenly whirled and went for the door, then turned back one last time with a self-satisfied grin and snarled, "Good-bye, sucker."

"Leo," I called after him.

"What?" he angrily replied.

"Would you do me a favor? Would you mind staying and finishing out the session?"

"What for?"

"You paid for it. You might as well stay."

"If you say so." Without looking at me, he sat down on the couch.

"Well, now what?" He was gazing at the floor, not at me.

"I felt really connected with you just now," I said. "I felt your realness. It made me care about you."

"Oh yeah?" His voice was half sarcastic and half grateful. He sighed deeply. "I don't believe you. You're just saying that. You're just interested in exploiting me like everyone else." He lay back on the couch, sighed again, and began to tremble. "Why should I believe you? Tell me one good reason why I should believe you." I didn't answer. He sighed one more time and began to shake as though some sudden gust of wind had enveloped him.

Leo then turned his head toward the wall, gasping mightily and holding his breath to prevent a small sob that finally broke through.

Chapter 5

Audrey:
Black Writing and White Writing

"I would say I'm a writer," she said. "Except that I'm not writing anything."

"Why aren't you writing?"

"I don't know what voice to use."

"What do you mean?"

"I don't know whether I'm writing for blacks or for whites. I don't know whether *I'm* black or white. I don't know who I am."

"That must be confusing."

"Must it? I'm not sure."

"You don't know who you really are?"

"Correct. I don't know who I am, and I don't know what I'm feeling."

"What are you feeling about me right now?"

"I don't know."

"Do you like me?"

"You seem nice, but I don't know if I like you."

"Do you hate me?"

"I don't know."

"Do you feel nervous about starting therapy?"

"No. I'm telling you, I don't know what I'm feeling."

"How long have you not known what you're feeling?"

"As long as I can remember."

Audrey sat before me wielding a wry, confident smile. To me and to the world in general she certainly appeared to have feelings and, in fact, at that moment her wry smile and direct gaze seemed to be alive with more than a little anger and bitterness. However, the rest of her—the matter-of-fact voice, the resigned chin, the downward face, the limp arms, the legs that were slightly apart, the conservative black dress that was draped over her like a blanket—contradicted that appearance, as though to say, "Don't believe what you see." Although physically she was an attractive woman, because of this underlying negation and its associated contraction of energy, she seemed to be missing some vital connection.

I gazed at her, sorting out what she had told me so far. She was in her late thirties and came from an educated African-American family. She had called me after she had tried working with several other therapists, none of whom had been able to "really understand" her. She did not know if any therapist could help her, especially a white one, but she was determined to give it one more try. She related a history of working obsessively at some job, climbing the ladder, and then suddenly one day not being able to get out of bed and go to her job. During the period that followed the quitting of a job, she would lie in her bed for days and feel nothing. She appeared to be manic-depressive, except for her claim not to know what she was feeling, a claim which I assumed was exaggerated.

"So," I said. "You don't know who you are?"

"I don't," she replied in a matter-of-fact manner, as though discussing the weather in her region. "I don't know who I am on a personal level. I only know who I am symbolically."

"And who are you symbolically?"

"I'm a black woman. I'm a black woman who has spent her life fighting racism in the public schools. I'm a symbol, you see; a symbol of the black struggle. I don't have a personality separate from that symbolism."

"But as a symbol you have feelings?"

She flashed the wry smile again. "Only anger about racism. That's it. That's all I'm allowed to be angry at."

"Allowed? By whom?"

"My father."

"I see. Are you aware of any anger at me, being that I'm a white therapist?"

"In that I have a generalized anger at whites, not to mention men, I could work up some anger at you on that symbolic level. On that symbolic level, because my mother was half white, I also have anger at blacks for their black racism toward whites, but not on a personal level. On a personal level I have no feelings. I pretend to have feelings; in my daily life I smile at people and show gobs of sympathy and love and understanding. I play the role of the virtuous, caring woman. My brother calls me Saint Audrey. He says I have a saint complex, whatever that means. I play the role magnificently and people tell me their problems and look up to me. But inside I know I'm faking. I don't know what I'm really feeling. It's all an act. Inside there's nothing but a void of confusion and despair."

Audrey, more than any other patient I have seen, fit the description of what Deutsch termed the "as if" personality type (Deutsch, 1942). In the early part of the twentieth century in Vienna, she met with a number of such personalities, young women who had dissociated or depersonalized to a point where they had no sense of any kind of identity, who went through life hiding behind a façade. Perhaps such young women were more prevalent during the Victorian era, when societal sexual repression was so all-encompassing. Deutsch saw these personalities as schizoid types, on the border of schizophrenia. Today they would probably be called borderlines.

Audrey had never developed a personality in the ordinary sense of that word. Her personality development had been arrested somewhere back in her early childhood. Hence, as an adult she did not know who she was. She had a finely honed façade, but her façade was unreal, not centered in her feelings. Hence, it was fragile. She did not possess a mature ego or a cohesive self. She suffered from identity confusion and low self-esteem, stemming from the sense of a void inside her (where her feelings should have been). Her ego could not adequately perform ordinary tasks such as reality testing, toleration of emotions, or delayed gratification. Her alienation from her self precluded her being able to achieve real intimacy with any individual and bound her destructively to her father. If people believed her false self and had positive feelings toward her, she despised them. If people did not believe her false self and had negative feelings toward her, she resented them. In addition, her identity diffusion prevented her from identifying herself as black or white or male or female, so that she did not feel comfortable with either blacks, whites, males, or females. She had spent her adult years in a virtual exile from herself and from others.

Her first therapist, to whom she went when she was about thirty, was a novice female who mirrored her false self; Audrey soon left her in contempt. Her second therapist, an African American, wanted to join her anger at whites, but he could not tolerate her anger at blacks or at her father. Her third therapist, a white male, did not believe in talking about the past, so he frustrated her need to analyze and reconstruct her childhood. It was at this point that she sought treatment with me. Her chief complaint was that she couldn't write.

"I used to be able to turn out stories that were touching in their way. That's when I was writing for *Black Wonder,* an African-American literary magazine," she told me early on in the treatment. "But then I developed this little conflict with the editors. They only wanted stories that portrayed blacks as victims. I had other ideas." She smiled with mock regret. "After I lost that job, I couldn't write anymore."

"What happens when you try to write?" I asked.

"I guess I don't know who I'm writing for. If I'm writing for blacks, then I have to adhere to certain rules, take a certain attitude, or else I'm regarded as a traitor to the black cause. If I'm writing for whites, there are completely different rules and a completely different attitude. I can never seem to say what I mean."

"We'll have to help you do that."

"Good luck."

She had brought me some stories she had written for *Black Wonder* and some other stories she had written for a white audience, and her conflict was apparent in those pieces. One of the stories that had appeared in *Black Wonder* was about a young African-American woman who had gone to a bank to get a college loan. When the bank turned down her loan application, she demanded to know why. "You don't have a credit rating," the manager told her. "You've never borrowed anything before, so we have no way of knowing if you're reliable." At first she felt the manager was being racist, and many in the black community where she lived encouraged her to take some kind of action against him. But then she met a young white woman who complained that she had been turned down for the same reason—because she had no credit rating. The story ended on an ambiguous note, with the protagonist sitting on a pier, unable to decide whether the bank was indeed racist. It did not seem to have a point of view, perhaps reflecting the fear and confusion in Audrey's own mind with regard to racial issues.

All creativity entails the risk of being truthful (most societies discourage the truth) or of doing something new and being repudiated for it, as May (1975) noted. But creative writing is probably the most risky of all. Writers have to put their point of view on the line in symbols—words—that are much more direct in their impact and clarity than the symbols in any other art form. A painting of a lover's quarrel is never as poignant or as specific or as detailed as a story, play, or movie of the same quarrel, and the point of view is much more evident. The writer of a novel can go inside a character's mind and make interpretations about what is being depicted: the woman thinking about how unfair life is and how she is continually exploited in relationships with men; the man thinking about how stupid the woman is and how stupid all women are; a chorus of relatives commenting on how the man and the woman are continually staging their quarrels at family gatherings. In the end it is quite apparent how the writer sees things.

When writers deal with a subject as controversial as racial and gender issues, viewpoint is all the more significant. If one is writing about an African-American man raping a European-American woman, the writer might take one of several perspectives. The writer might write from the point of view of the man, viewing him as a victim of the system of white prejudice and privilege, of which the woman partakes. Or the writer might write from the perspective of the woman, portraying her as a victim of the male system of prejudice and privilege, of which the man partakes. Each of these points of view is biased. The most universal point of view would be to write with an omniscient voice—as if one were from Mars and were looking at the incident with a completely fresh understanding and profound insight into the various underlying motivations of both the man and woman and their cultural backgrounds. However, most of what is called art is biased—and hence, a partisan ideology.

From the time humans could communicate, they have been involved in ideological conflicts. At one moment or another an ideology becomes dominant and censors all others. In certain countries, the Catholic ideology predominates, while in others it is the communist ideology. In some it is the sociologist, and in others, the fascist. In American society, we have many ideological conflicts on political, racial, gender, and religious lines. In addition, there are also ideological debates in the various fields, such as art. As I write this, you may be questioning the statements I'm making about ideology and about the nature of creative writing. If I were writing about racial subjects, you would probably have your own ideas, strong ones, about race, which would cause you to question each statement I made about race. Almost everybody who writes enters this ideological cross-current, like it or not. One can take any of several fashionable positions, or become enmeshed in fear and indecision, because that personal and cultural issues have collided internally, creating an impasse.

Audrey's writer's block could be studied on several levels. On the surface, it seemed to be a product of the racial and sexual cultural climate that prevailed in America at that time. Below that level, her writer's block appeared to be linked to a racial identity conflict; she couldn't write because she didn't know who she was. However, when Audrey and I analyzed her identity conflict, we uncovered myriad associations and memories about her childhood, in which she had been constantly in the middle in numerous ways.

Audrey was a middle child, caught between two half-brothers. The older brother was the offspring of her father and his first wife, who died during labor. The younger brother was the offspring of her father's third wife, Audrey's stepmother. Her father was African American with dark skin. Her mother, who was of mixed race (her mother's mother had been white and her father had been part black and part Native American), had lighter skin. Audrey resembled her mother in both figure and skin color, while her brothers had the darker skin of their father.

She did not see much of her father during her first three years. He developed an illness and was in and out of the hospital, and for a time it appeared he might die. During that period she recalled being close to her mother. Her earliest memory was about an incident of urinary incontinence: she wet her pants while at nursery school and felt horrified by it. Her mother was "very kind" and told her, "Those things happen." She recalled feeling love for her mother. Sometime around the same year, her father came home from the hospital and began a long convalescence. At first he seemed like a stranger, and Audrey was afraid of him.

Soon after he came home an event occurred which was pivotal to her childhood development. One night she heard her mother and father quarreling. She wobbled sleepily into their bedroom to find her mother aiming a pistol at her father—the same pistol her father kept in a drawer beside the bed. As Audrey stood in the doorway, the gun went off, wounding her father in the shoulder. Her mother later explained that she and Audrey's father were having an argument about which school Audrey was going to attend the following year. Her father, who was a minister, wanted to send her to an all-white school in order to force the school to integrate. Her mother was absolutely against it, saying she did not want her daughter to be used in this way. Their feelings about this issue were quite strong, and her father was stubborn about his right, as the father, to decide the matter.

Her mother was convicted of assault but did not serve any time in prison. Instead, she agreed to divorce Audrey's father and to giving up custody of Audrey. She also agreed not to see Audrey again. Hence, at the age of five, Audrey was separated from her mother and did not see her again until Audrey was an adult. She recalled going to the train station with her mother on the day she packed her things and left, clinging tightly to her, asking why she couldn't go with her. "Please don't leave me," she begged. "Please, please, please don't leave me, Mommy. Please. Let me go with you. Why can't I go with you?" She did not want to stay with her father, who was still a stranger to her.

"You have to stay," said Audrey's mother. "The court said so. I can't do anything about it. But I'll always be thinking of you, and I'll always love you."

As Audrey returned to the house with her father and older brother, she felt terrified, knowing her father had seen her beg her mother to take her away. From then on, she believed she had to be extra careful to please her father, lest he exact revenge on her for being "a traitor."

It became her task to care for him during his convalescence. This care included bathing him. Until she had shot him, his wife had done this bathing, but afterward he did not want her to touch him and enlisted Audrey to take over this chore. She recalled seeing her father's penis and wanting to touch it (he washed his own penis), and had many erotic, oedipal fantasies about being her father's wife and having his children. After the session when she recalled this memory, she brought in a dream that alluded to this period. In the dream, she was masturbating a horse or some kind of four-legged animal. It had a dog's penis, but the animal was bigger than a dog. When I asked for her associations to this dream, she recalled bathing her father and seeing his penis. I interpreted her confusion about what kind of animal she was masturbating to the confused feelings she must have had about bathing her father—a mixture of resentment about being taken away from her mother, erotic excitement at winning her father and being privy to such intimacy with him, guilt about crossing the incest taboo, and perhaps a fear and envy of this appendage, which she and her mother did not possess, and which left them both helpless under its power. In addition, the horse and dog may have symbolized her feeling that her father was an "animal."

Soon afterward, her father remarried a woman who was much like her mother, but much younger. From the time the stepmother appeared, any semblance of intimacy with her father ceased completely. Indeed, her stepmother quickly intervened and would not allow Audrey to even talk with her father, asserting that, "He's busy, don't bother him." Her relationship with her stepmother was quite strained. She described the latter as being competitive and jealous of her, flaunting her sexual relationship with her father by kissing him and sitting on his lap in front of the children, acting like a child herself.

At this time her father began sending her to all-white schools. Each fall they would move to a new town, and he would send her to a new school. As a black minister, he would make pronouncements in each district about the evils of segregation, defiantly bringing his older son and daughter to each new school, usually accompanied by federal marshals. Audrey remembered the isolation of being the only black student in each school, but also the sense of moral superiority at having all of these white students hate her and feeling pity for them. She recalled moving from town to town, feeling isolated, never being able to make any friends, black or white, never being able to make any lasting attachments other than those to her own immediate family.

"That must have been when I developed my Saint Audrey persona," she remarked, upon recalling this period. "My father would always preach that my brother and I should only have love and pity for the white students. We weren't supposed to have any hatred for anybody. We were supposed to be above it all. However, we could see that this was a case of 'Do as I say, not as I do' for it was quite evident that he had tons of anger toward whites. So, on a verbal level we were told not to have anger at whites, while his own behavior told us that in actuality it was allowable."

What was definitely not allowed was to have any anger—or any complaint whatsoever—about her father or her stepmother. She was expected to be a good girl, who did as she was told and never uttered a contradictory word, and she tried her best to be that girl, but it was impossible. Her father had a temper, and she could never predict when that temper would flare or what conduct would be found wanting. She recalled that on one occasion, when the family was to meet at a cemetery to pay it's respects to a deceased aunt, she and her brother decided they did not want to go, so they stayed home. When her father and stepmother returned from the cemetery, they were furious at this disobedience and he whipped both of them. His way of whipping them was unique: he would have them lie on their beds, place a pillow over their heads and sit on them so they could not move or scream. Then he would give them 100 whacks. If he heard them scream, he would yell, "Swallow it." This way of punishment, termed by Miller (1983) as "poisonous pedagogy," ensures that a child will be severely disturbed emotionally, with a tendency to suppress anger.

As she became more disturbed and more isolated in the family, she developed a reputation as the family oddball. Her brothers teased her about being oversensitive. Her stepmother saw her as a threat and condescended to her. She was the only girl, the daughter of a woman whom her father never talked about, the child with lighter skin. She perceived a double standard in the way her brothers were treated and the way she was treated by her father and by her paternal grandmother, who would visit frequently and dote on her father and her brothers but be contemptuous toward her. There was apparently a generational pattern in the family of showing extreme favoritism toward sons and contempt toward daughters.

One of the dreams she brought into therapy during the initial stage shows her conflicting feelings about her family. She was on a boat with her father, brothers, and stepmother. Suddenly they disappeared. The boat moved along a river, and on the bank she saw statues of Greek gods, all toppled over. Then she realized her family was still there but asleep. She woke them and asked, "Did you see that?" "No," they answered. "We didn't see anything." She told them to look back, but they couldn't see the statues. The dream not only indicates her idealization (her family as Greek gods), but also her anger in the form of a wish for them to disappear (as they do in the beginning), or at least to be knocked off their pedestals. The fact that she could see something that they couldn't see denotes her need to repress and deny her family's aggression toward her, as well as her family's continual misunderstanding of her. It also shows her alienation from them (she is the oddball in the dream, as in real life).

From the time she went off to college and later when she lived by herself in New York, she had had only brief relationships with men. She would give herself to them sexually, feeling nothing for them, enjoying no sexual pleasure, and then not see them again. She related to them as a saint, as Saint Audrey, listening to them, controlling them, keeping them at a distance, thereby maintaining a sense of superiority. Relationships with women were nonexistent—her competitive urges sabotaged all attempts. Intellectually gifted, she would excel at jobs for a year or two, then be unable to continue. The one secondary gratification that sustained her was her narcissistic belief in her own innate superiority—an intellectual and moral superiority—and she clung to this belief as a child clings to a security blanket. This secret delusion compensated for her exile: she was alone, she told herself, because she was too good for the world, too good for blacks, too good for whites. Hence, no one could understand her, including her string of therapists.

When she was thirty-five years old, this delusion of superiority and control was shattered. She had met a man whom she thought was different from the rest, whom she thought was on her level. He was a black man, but one with class. He was a businessman with an air of confidence and determination that attracted her to him. They saw each other for a few months, and he seemed to understand her like nobody else had ever understood her. He understood her the way she wanted to be understood: "You're a saint," he told her. "A savvy saint. You pretend you're beneath everybody, but in fact you know more than everyone." This was music to her ears, following on the heels of the critical messages she had gotten from her family. She opened up to him, even felt sexual pleasure, and entertained thoughts of marrying him. Then, on that pivotal day, she received a bank statement indicating that her $30,000 in savings, which she had been planning to use for law school, had been withdrawn. The man had disappeared, and she was never able to find him. She had lost him, her money, and her false self, with its fragile sense of superiority.

When news got out of her humiliation, her father, her stepmother, and her two brothers all deserted her. She was an embarrassment to the family, and they wanted nothing to do with her. At about that time, she had a recurring dream in which she found her family dead—her father, stepmother, and two brothers. She did not know how they had died, but she buried them in a pit. Somehow she could see through the dirt, as if she had X-ray vision, and saw rats eating their bodies. This dream was a puzzlement to her, for in her waking life, she continued to view things from her family's perspective and didn't harbor any anger toward them. If they deserted her now, she decided, they probably had a good reason. She was the bad one.

When therapists encourage patients to work through their feelings about their parents and siblings—to feel the anger, hurt, fear and the like—it is in order to foster the individuation and the separation process. It is quite common for people like Audrey to continue to use their family as their reference group and to see themselves as their family sees them. Only when they have felt their real feelings and distinguished between how their family sees them and how they actually see themselves and their families, can they regain an authentic sense of who they are.

As her therapy progressed, we were able to understand how her writer's block was linked not only to her confusion about her racial identity, but also to her confusion about her family allegiance (should she be loyal to her father or her mother? Should she think "male" or "female"?), to her role as "racial symbol" in all-white schools, and to her position as middle child in her family. However, on the surface, in her present life, the block was related to an inability to know her feelings or to perceive life realistically. Obviously, if one cannot perceive life realistically, one cannot write realistically.

This latter difficulty showed itself prominently during the first year of therapy. After the "honeymoon" was over, she began to view me, unrealistically, as somebody who was not to be trusted. I was at times her father, to be revered but feared and, unconsciously, hated; at times her older or younger brothers, whom she resented; and at other times her mother, who would be tender and caring but who might abandon her. In any case, I was an exalted figure. This meant that she idealized me and needed my approval and my permission to exist. This also meant she hated me.

When she was angry at something I had said or done, she would verbalize generalized anger at whites. "I was sitting on the bus today and a white man was sitting next to me. He had his legs all spread out as if he were the only one on the bus, and I wished I had had a knife and could stab him in the knee," she said one day. Knowing she was really talking about me, I encouraged her to continue. She went on a tirade about white men and their imperial attitudes.

"I know what you mean," I replied, being very careful to mirror her point of view. It was not that I thought she was entirely wrong. Racism does exist. However, her narcissistic need to make racism responsible for all her problems and the allied refusal to take any responsibility for her own contribution to her bad relationships and to minimize the contribution of her dysfunctional family complicated the transference. Elsewhere (Schoenewolf, 1993) I have written about this kind of resistance, which I call a "cultural resistance" because it originates from the cultural climate in society as well as from the family environment. During this time, I became a symbol of white oppression or of white male oppression. Because of this, occasional impasses developed during which she became so furious at me and so convinced that, as a white male, I could not understand her, she would fall silent.

My way of breaking this impasse was to insist that she see me as a human being, not as male or white. As simple as this sounds, it turned out not to be so simple at all. During the time of this treatment, issues of sexism and racism were in the news daily, and it was difficult for blacks and whites or men and women to disregard each other's gender or skin color and relate to each other as humans. Ironically, the very emphasis on issues of gender and race heightened one's focus on gender and race and increased the polarity. Yet I persisted.

"The only way we're going to get past this impasse is to forget about politics and concentrate on what you're feeling and what I'm feeling. It's important for you to distinguish between your assumptions about me as a symbolic white male, and the reality of how I'm actually acting toward you in the here and now. Am I trying to oppress you? Is my attitude negative or demeaning? Am I making any stereotypical assumptions about you?"

"There's nothing I can really pinpoint, except for your having me lie on the couch while you sit up. It's rather oppressive. It places me in a subservient position."

"I've tried to explain that this is the way that fosters the deepest kind of change. I'm not asking you to do anything I haven't done myself."

"That sounds right. But I'm still not sure I can trust you. You may just be pretending for the sake of the treatment. I don't know how you behave outside these walls when you see a black person. For all I know, you may be two-faced, like all the whites I've ever met." After going over this again and again, she eventually came to realize that it was she, rather than I, who had been making the stereotypical assumptions.

Resolving this cultural resistance was a turning point in the therapy. Once she understood that I was not The White Male but a human being with his own unique thoughts and feelings, it became easier to work on material related to her father, brothers, and mother and the many resistances associated with it. As we did this, her repression of her real feelings and memories began to pry loose. The displacement of her rage onto me and onto whites and men gave way to a more complicated picture of feelings and memories about her father, mother, brothers, and other people in her life. At the same time, the transference toward me became more characterological than cultural, rooted in an oral-stage merger with me as a surrogate mother.

Her negative feelings about me reached a high point when she called me to cancel a session, and I failed to return her call promptly. She came in angry the following session and lay silently on the couch for about five minutes. When she finally spoke, she said she felt too dependent on me and regretted that she had opened up to me so much. She remembered a time during her childhood when another girl was living with her family. She thought the other girl was her friend and confided in her one day that she hated her stepmother because she was cruel to her. The girl then went to Audrey's parents and told them what she had said. Her parents punished Audrey severely for this, calling her a traitor for telling a non-family member such things. Never once did her parents inquire why she was so unhappy with the stepmother. I interpreted that she had had originally repressed this memory and it had now been rekindled due to the transference.

Audrey then recalled a recent happening. She was riding in a car with her father and stepmother. Her stepmother said nothing to her during the whole ride, ignoring her, talking only to Audrey's father, as was her custom. Then she turned around and said, "Audrey, honey, I've noticed that you have a habit of saying 'you know.' Do you realize how that sounds when you keep saying 'you know, you know, you know?' It's very immature." For the rest of the trip, Audrey found herself uttering "you know" even more.

"I don't normally say 'you know.' The reason I was saying 'you know' in the first place was because my parents, particularly my stepmother, make me nervous. And then for her to pounce on that phrase was like adding insult to injury."

"Yes, it was," I told her.

"I'm glad you're here," she said, smiling back toward me. "I think I would have gone crazy without you."

Going into her third year of therapy, Audrey began to be an analytic patient. Her ego was finally strong enough to tolerate interpretations and make use of them. She revived more and more memories, made more connections with the present, and improved her coping skills. We forged an effective therapeutic alliance and that enabled us to reconstruct her childhood, and analyze the transference and resistance. As we did all of this, she regained her ability to write. This happened gradually.

With Audrey, I used almost exclusively analytic introspection. There was a lot of painstaking analytic work before she found her own voice—many dreams that needed to be gone over numerous times; long hours of excavating memories and working through them; and the delicate and emotional analyzing of her transferences to me as well as the accompanying resistance to the process. When she found her voice, it was neither a black voice nor a white voice—nor a particularly female voice. It reflected neither her father's nor her mother's attitude. It was a "middle" voice, one that distinctively saw both sides of things—including both sides of the black-white racial conflict—and did so in an authoritative manner with empathy for both sides.

She got around to revising the story about the young woman who wanted a college loan. In the revised version, the young woman's monologue, upon getting turned down, takes over the story. The narrator's reflections about race, African-American culture, her family, and the politics of race, filled several pages and were, in and of themselves, the purpose and meaning of the story. In the earlier version, her voice was confused or nonexistent; now it was rich with feeling and a confident sense of who she was and how she saw things.

At one time Audrey had thought that being in the middle meant she was wishy-washy, but now she had come to see it as a strength—as a special ability to be objective about issues that are so often nowadays fraught with hysteria.

Chapter 6

Jerome and Betty:
The Musician and the Painter
Who Needed to Suffer

Suffering, according to an old folk saying, purifies the soul. I would amend that saying: Suffering that has been understood and processed purifies the soul. Many artists believe in a variation of the first saying, harboring the notion that suffering alone purifies the artistic vision.

Jerome was a young man in his late twenties who harbored this notion about musicians. "To be a musician, you have to suffer," he would repeat like a mantra. "It comes with the territory. If you want to be a musician or any kind of artist, you suffer. Period."

During his first year of therapy, Jerome had spent much of the time explaining in vivid detail the many ways he had suffered as a musician and as a person. "You don't know what it's like in the music world," he would note in a voice tinged with resignation. "They treat you like an animal. There's so much pettiness, so much manipulation, so much vanity. I'd like to just do my music and not have to worry about politics, but if you want to get ahead, you've got to make contacts." What riled him most was that other people were better at making contacts. "I found out today that George Bollinger got a fifty-thousand-dollar deal from Atlantic. I used to jam with him. He's a total poseur. He's got a pretty face, and that's all. But that's what they want these days."

Several times a month, Jerome's mother would call him and tell him how well his younger brother was doing in medical school. His mother had been telling him how well his younger brother had been doing ever since he had been born, which was four years after his own birth. She had told him how well his younger brother had first walked and how nicely he went to the potty. ("You didn't go to the potty until you were two-and-a-half," she reminded him.) Later, she cackled over how industrious the younger brother was, and she crooned over how popular the brother was in high school and how he excelled in sports and how he made the honor roll. ("You never made the honor roll, did you?" she would ask him from time to time.) In despair, he retreated into his own world, a world filled with music—his one great love. He sublimated all his frustration into music, and music in turn became an obsession. Now, as a young adult, he still heard from his mother about how well his younger brother was doing; yet he seldom spoke of his mother or his younger brother during his psychotherapy sessions.

"I wish I could explain to you how it is in the New York music scene," he would repeat like a broken CD. "I mean, I know my music is good. I just know it. But that's not enough. You need to be a politician. Like George Bollinger and all the rest of the no-talent jerks." He looked at me with his dark, brooding eyes.

"And your brother?" I threw in. "What about him?"

"What about him?"

"Is he a politician?"

He laughed bitterly. "Funny you should mention him. Yes, the ultimate politician. He could always get anything he wanted from my mother. Anything. But I don't want to talk about him. That's all in the past. Fuck him. What really ticks me off are the no-talent jerks walking around with their electric . . . bongos! I mean, I can't go through a single day without running into one of them, and they all think they're so superior to me. They all think they're musical geniuses." He looked at me from the corners of his eyes. "Do you know what I'm saying?"

"Yes, I understand," I said. Like many patients, he had a tendency to want to maintain his repression of the psychological traumas of the past and to transfer the feelings from those past relationships onto the present ones. The aversive circumstances that had permeated his childhood had shaped his personality in such a way that he no longer had the capacity to adapt to present circumstances. My job was to encourage him to put those feelings back where they belonged and process them, so that they wouldn't influence his present situation. "But I was just wondering about your brother. I know it's in the past, but I was just wondering whether you are aware of still feeling any anger at him or at your mother."

"I don't know. Yeah, I remember once yelling at my mother, and she said to me, "Don't you ever raise your voice to me like that again. We could always give you away, you know."

"What did you say then?"

"I don't know. Nothing, probably. My mother had this thing about being a good mother. She never wanted to hear anything that suggested she wasn't a good mother. If you said anything at all like that she'd treat you as though you were a traitor. She was always telling me I was over-reacting or that I was oversensitive. Do you think I'm oversensitive?" Before I could answer, he answered his own question, as was his custom. "Sure, I'm oversensitive. It's the price you pay for being an artist. To be an artist is to suffer. Artists have to suffer because of their sensitivity; you see what I mean? But I'm not talking about these no-talent jerks. They don't suffer. I'm talking about real artists. Look at all the artists, writers, and musicians who went mad, who lived tragic lives."

Artistic suffering. Again and again he would come back to that. Month after month he would explain about the music scene and suffering and artistic sensitivity. Now and then I would venture a question, an interpretation, a gesture, but the patient did not seem interested in what I thought; he was more interested in explaining about art and suffering so that I could understand it. He wanted me to be a narcissistic extension of himself—or, as Kohut (1971) put it, a "selfobject" which would ally itself with his idealized self and look appreciatively at all he said (this is what he had needed from his mother when he was a toddler, as all children do). For a long time I had to do just that, until his ego was strong enough to tolerate more objectivity.

Over the years I have had numerous patients who have had this notion that their suffering was necessary for the production of art, and who were unable to distinguish between artistic sensitivity and neurotic sensitivity. Some, like Jerome, stayed with therapy and eventually were able to reframe how they saw things and change their self-defeating attitude. Others, like Betty, were so adamant that their neurosis was essential to their creativity that they left therapy abruptly in order to prevent me from tampering with their talent.

Betty, a talented painter, came to me because she was in an abusive relationship with an older man. She had had an abusive relationship with her parents, and now as an adult she had gone through a series of abusive relationships with men. Since she had no real connection with other people, all of her libido was sublimated into her painting. Nothing mattered to her except her art.

"All I really want," she would say over an over, "is to be left alone."

"Won't you be lonely if you're left alone?"

"Not at all. I've been alone all my life. Why do I need people? All they do is bother me. I just want to paint."

She was a thin, nervous young woman who painted thin, nervous old women—her mother, her aunts, friends of her mothers. Why she specialized in painting these old women with sad faces most likely had to do with the maternal deprivation she had suffered as a child. She had been an unwanted child whose parents did not even take a photograph of her until she was about twelve years old. Her paintings of sad old women were her way of dealing with the sadness inside her; through her portraits she could somehow objectify that sadness and place it at its source: her mother and her mother's sad, peasant existence.

As a child, Betty tried to be her mother's therapist, listening to the latter's rants about her father and being sympathetic to her mother's hard life. Betty hoped that by doing so, her mother would come around and be able to give her the love she needed. That had never happened. Now, in turning out the paintings of sad old women, she could continue to display sympathy for her mother's—and other women's—struggles and thereby sustain the unconscious hope for her own salvation. It was an irrational hope that somehow through these paintings she could illuminate and justify in her mind the fact that her mother, her aunts, and other women hadn't been able to give her the attention she needed. Through therapy, she came to understand and acknowledge this hope.

Her interest in therapy, however, was only marginal. She came because she was in a crisis about her husband. After she had left him and the therapy sessions were less about him and more about her, she began to see me as she saw everybody else: someone who was bothering her and standing as an obstacle to her pursuit of painting. Like Jerome, she was obsessed with making it as an artist, viewing artistic success as her vindication as a human being. While supporting herself by doing freelance work, she devoted all her spare time to painting, to taking her slides to galleries, to inviting gallery directors to her studio, and to attending art openings.

"I don't think I can afford therapy any more," she would often say. I knew that she could afford it. Invariably, when patients use money as an excuse for quitting therapy, deeper issues lie underneath, which they don't want to know about or disclose. I've noticed that, in most cases, when people really want to do something, they'll find the money for it.

"Putting the money issue aside, how are you feeling about therapy?"

"I think it's helped me a lot, but right now I have too many other things to do."

"But therapy is only one hour a week."

"I know, but I have to interrupt my painting to come here, and I don't like to interrupt my painting."

"So you see me as somebody who's distracting you, just like the other people in your life."

"Sort of. I know you support me, but yes, you do distract me."

"What else? What else am I trying to do?"

"Well, the only thing I can think of is that you don't really understand me. You keep trying to get me to relax and let go. You want me to remember the past and cry, and I don't think that will do any good. I've already cried about my past. My parents and I have a different relationship now. They're beginning to accept me. And anyway, I need my creative tension. It's what motivates me to paint. If you take away my tension, I'll have nothing. What will I be then? Who will I be?"

This was the refrain she always "sang" to me when I encouraged her to talk about her feelings about therapy. I would try to make her see how her tension was destructive to her. "Your creative tension, as you call it, may be motivating you, but it's motivating you in the wrong way. It's a form of vindication; your very salvation as a person rests on your achieving success as an artist. That puts a lot of pressure on you, and it also affects the kind of art you produce. Instead of being a vindication, it should be a relaxing, enjoyable form of play."

Betty would interrupt me, focusing only on one phrase. "I don't think it affects the kind of art I produce. You sound just like my mother. She can't understand why I'm always painting old women. That's what I choose to paint. That's what's inside of me. I have no choice but to paint them!"

"I think your paintings of old women are wonderful. I'm just saying that your reason for painting them creates a lot of tension inside of you that is destructive. At the deepest layer of your unconscious, the reason why you're painting is so that you can get love. So that you can get the love you never got from your parents." I knew that she would not be able to take in this interpretation now, but I also knew that she'd be out of the door soon, and I hoped that perhaps at some future point the words would have meaning to her. "But right now in your life you're rejecting everybody who wants to love you, including me. We're all a bother. By pushing everybody away, by nurturing isolation rather than intimacy, by maintaining a high state of tension because you think it's essential to your motivation, you're making yourself sicker. You're constantly in a state of discontent because you're convinced you can only be happy after you've achieved success. But if you pin all your hopes on success, how do you think you'll be able to handle that success once you achieve it?"

"I know, I know. I need to relax more. You're right. But it's hard to relax here in New York, with people constantly bothering me. I can't go on the subway without some man bothering me. I just wish I could go away and do my art."

Betty left therapy, despite my objections, just at the point when she had been accepted by a Soho gallery. She had a successful one-person show titled, "Farm Women," and sold six paintings for $10,000 each, earning more in a few weeks than she had earned in several years of working as a freelancer. In addition, her work had garnered critical praise in a few prestigious art magazines and great word of mouth. Her paintings were declared "feminist visions," and she was made into a feminist icon.

I called Betty to congratulate her on her success and ask how she was. "I'm fine," she replied in a rather perfunctory way. "I'm doing well. Have you seen my latest show? I've thought about you sometimes. Maybe I'll come back to therapy one of these days. Anyway, it's good to hear from you." When I pressed her about how she was really doing, she admitted that she had had migraine headaches for several weeks, had recently broken up with another unavailable man, and was smoking marijuana from the time she got up in the morning to the time she went to bed late at night.

"Perhaps you should come in for a follow-up session," I suggested.

"I'll think about it."

Unfortunately, she never did.

Therapy is a profession that can be wearing if you allow yourself to become too involved. You have to be able to accept that there are people you can help and people you can't help, and in order make that distinction you must work through your own issues (the conscious and the unconscious issues) so that they don't affect your therapy relationships. Betty, sadly, was someone I couldn't help. Jerome, on the other hand, eventually came around.

It took several years, but finally, in the middle of one of his long explanatory obloquies, he ran out of words. He had been talking, as usual, about suffering and artistic sensitivity and how he needed it for his creative well-being—but not with the usual degree of certainty. In fact, after only a few minutes, he came to a halt and sat glancing at me uneasily, an expression of confusion on his face. He was silent for a while.

"What's going on?" I asked.

"I was just wondering . . . what you think."

"What I think about what?"

"I was wondering . . . what you think about suffering and sensitivity, wondering if you think . . . artists are more sensitive than the average person?"

It was the first time he had ever allowed me to be anything but a "yes man." I knew this signaled that he had transcended his narcissistic mode and had stepped upon the threshold of mature object-relations. However, I kept the discussion on an abstract level, sensing that he might not be able to handle anything too direct. Slowly and deliberately I pointed out to him the distinction, as I saw it, between artistic sensitivity and neurotic sensitivity. I spoke at some length about how artistic sensitivity was a positive quality that served to make artists more attuned to things such as truth and beauty. It was something you were born with—eyes that could see color and form; ears that could hear sounds in harmony; hearts that could feel the pulse of the unconscious. I compared an artist to a finely tuned instrument such as a microscope that could see to the depth of things (purposely trying to feed the patient's grandiosity in order that he might listen to the next part of the explanation).

"Yes, yes, I know what you're saying," he shot in, nodding with enthusiasm.

I went on somewhat solemnly. "This kind of sensitivity, artistic sensitivity, does involve some suffering, but it's a different kind of suffering than neurotic suffering. It's the kind of suffering you feel when you have a bitter-sweet insight into life's preciousness and finiteness, or the labor pains of composing some new, original harmony that you know won't be understood by most others.

"Neurotic sensitivity, on the other hand, is the cause of a great deal of suffering that prevents artists from using their artistic sensitivity and fulfilling themselves. Neurotic sensitivity is an overreaction to one's present life circumstances due to unresolved conflicts in the past." To illuminate this point, I created a story about a woman who had a younger sister who was always considered by their father to be prettier than she was, so that all her life the woman felt inferior to her sister and jealous of her and neurotically sensitive to remarks about her appearance. She was always suffering because of her feelings of inferiority. I watched Jerome closely as I related this story and his eyes appeared quite thoughtful. I assumed I was reaching him. "So you see," I concluded, "you don't have to suffer to be an artist. Not the way you're suffering. If anything, suffering blocks you from realizing your full potential."

There was a meditative silence. Then the patient sat up in his chair with a wide-eyed expression, nodding slowly as though a dawning were taking place somewhere among the dendrites of his brain.

"Yes, yes, I know exactly what you're saying," he replied animatedly. "That's exactly what I've been trying to explain to you. I'm not oversensitive like my mother thinks; I have artistic sensitivity. I'm not using my artistic sensitivity though, and so I have to suffer. Oh, well, it's a good thing I have my music. I don't know what I'd do without my music. It's everything to me. Everything."

I was a bit disappointed, thinking that once again I had not reached him. However, the first thing he asked when he came in for his next session was, "So you think I'm suffering because I'm *neurotic,* is that it?"

Chapter 7

Norbert:
The Filmmaker Who Couldn't Finish

Norbert entered treatment soon after he had received his MFA in film from a prestigious graduate school in the East. He had almost not graduated because he hadn't been able to complete his final project, a full-length film, which he was to write and direct. However, his professor liked him—he had been an industrious student in all other ways—and allowed him to turn in his partially completed film along with a synopsis of the rest of it for complete credit. He was now making his living working on the crews of whatever movie was being filmed in New York.

"It's tough working on these crews," he would say as he lay on my couch, "because I'm always thinking that the script's inept and I, of course, could write a better one, or the director's vision is inferior to my own. But then when I sit down to write a script, everything I write seems abysmally flawed." As he spoke he had a smirk on his face. This smirk, which was almost always lurking somewhere around his mouth, was a defensive posture, as if he needed to say to others what he anticipated they would think of him: "Don't be ridiculous! You can't write a film! You can't even write a grammatically correct sentence." He was a tall, gangly young man with a decidedly intellectual persona, whose grammar was in fact superior. Indeed, early in his therapy he had corrected my pronunciation of the word "lambaste"—pointing out that the second syllable rhymed with "haste"—to my slight embarrassment.

Because of his analytic bent, he would often ask me for my analysis of his situation. "What do you think my problem is?"

"You have an inferiority/superiority conflict," I told him. "You can't make up your mind if you're inferior or superior. And that's because it's a double bind. Being inferior is, of course, painful; but being superior is threatening. When you come across as inferior, people treat you that way, and that's no fun. But if you assert your superiority, people want to knock you down. So you're paralyzed."

"I think you're right. That's exactly it; I hide behind my aura of inferiority, terrified to assert myself. I *am* paralyzed in just about every way. I'm paralyzed as a filmmaker, and I'm also paralyzed sexually. I don't know whether to be homosexual or heterosexual. The former orientation seems inferior to me, and the latter seems superior and threatening. I hate everything about the gay scene; it seems so effete and pathetic. But if I try to be heterosexual, I feel like a poseur, and I'm afraid I'm going to be found out and knocked down by straight men or by straight women. I can't win."

"So it would appear." He had a penchant for taking my interpretations and running with them, perhaps to demonstrate his superior analytical skills. However, I have learned that the more people figure things out for themselves, the faster the therapy proceeds. After he had added his own interpretation to mine, he would always sigh and shake his head.

"My God, that all sounds terrible."

"It *is* a bind."

"Help," he replied. "How do I get out of it?"

"By talking about it."

Gradually, smirkingly, he told me his story. Norbert was another of the many patients who had to serve as a selfobject for a narcissistic parent—in this case his mother. He was designated as the child who would mirror her the way she wanted to be mirrored. She wanted to believe that she was a perfectly wise and good mother and wife who did everything for her husband and children and got little credit for it. She wanted to believe that she was a superior human who had married beneath her. She was from an upper-class background; her husband was from a lower-class background. She liked the finer things—books, art, music—while he was content to sit in front of the television set and watch football games, drink beer, and read the financial report. She would "work her fingers to the bone," in order to see that the children had a cooked, nutritious meal every night, clean and ironed clothes, and were caught up on their homework. He barely noticed what was going on with the children. She was the martyr, her husband the slob. This was her vision of things, and this also became Norbert's vision.

Norbert, her second-oldest son, quickly learned to understand her the way she wanted to be understood. He supported her completely. He was an almost exact mirror of her ego ideal. He had to be. If he ever slipped and did not mirror her correctly, if he, for instance, questioned something such as, "But Mother, maybe it's not necessary for you to cook three separate meals tonight to fit the schedules of everybody, especially since you have a headache and are feeling rundown," he was doomed.

"Yes, it *is* necessary," she would snap back. "If I don't do it, who will? Do you think your father would ever lift a finger around here? Don't tell me what to do. You sound just like your father when you talk like that. Just help me set the table or shut up and get out of my way!"

He never knew when his mother would, as he put it, "turn on me." She was constantly sending him double messages. For example, she would continually complain about Norbert's father, saying, "He acts like a man; what can I say!" Norbert, trying to be in perfect harmony, applied himself all the harder toward becoming a feminine man. Then one day, in speaking of a timid neighbor, she spat out, "I hate domesticated men." Devastated by such inconsistencies, he would strive even harder to stay one step ahead of her, despite her unpredictability. Even on her deathbed—she died of cancer in middle-age—he continued to be the dutiful son, swallowing all his own hurt, rage, guilt, and jealousy, suppressing his real self in order to tell her once again that she had been the perfect mother and wife whose nobility had been tragically unappreciated. By that time he had begun therapy, but he couldn't get himself to tell her about it, for he was sure she would view therapy as a disguised attack on her parenting.

Norbert was born into an environment in which attention was scant. Norbert's older brother, three years his senior, was a blue-eyed, blond-haired kid named Will. His mother called Will "a spoiled brat." Compared to Will, Norbert always felt like an ugly duckling, with his brown hair, brown eyes, and skinny, awkward frame. Their mother had tried to train Will to be a selfobject, but he had turned down the role and seemed stubbornly intent on being a troublemaker instead. His father and mother spent a good deal of their time fighting over how to deal with Will's bad behavior; meanwhile, Norbert felt invisible from birth onward. Seeing that his older brother was a problem because of his rebelliousness against his parents, especially his mother, Norbert resolved early to be the exact opposite of his brother. This gave him another reason to please his mother in every way—another reason to never assert himself at all—since even the mildest form of self-assertion seemed like rebellion.

His mother had seven children, spaced about a year and a half apart. Thus she had her third child, a girl, at a time when Norbert was amid what Mahler, Pine, and Bergman (1975) refer to as the anal-rapprochement phase. This is a very difficult phase for a child, in which he or she has to complete three developmental tasks: potty training, separation from mother, and the formation of gender identity. We speculated that his potty training must have been too early and must have left him feeling dirty and ashamed (adding to his inferiority complex). His separation-individuation never really happened, and his gender identity formation—the process in which a boy discovers the two sexes and identifies himself as distinctly male—was put on hold. Shengold (1989) added another layer of understanding to this phase when he expanded on the classical notion that anality is connected with narcissism (grandiosity compensating for the shameful act of soiling) and served as a defense against ego loss. This seemed particularly true with Norbert, for whom anality was a continual theme in his dreams and in his life.

"I had another attack of diarrhea last night," Norbert would frequently confess in his sessions.

"What happened yesterday?" I would ask.

"I guess I must have been stressed out."

Invariably his bouts of diarrhea followed days in which he had asserted himself in some way and felt terrified because of it. The act of defecation was symbolic—so it seemed—of his "dirtiness" or inferiority, as well as his harmlessness as a male (representing a regression to a rather helpless and infantile mode). Similar to his smirk, the diarrhea had a defensive purpose; it was an attempt to ward off any possible attacks on his personality by announcing to the world: Look, don't you see? I'm beneath you; I'm dirty; I'm harmless.

As Norbert became older he was enlisted as "assistant caretaker," helping his mother tend the two girls who followed him. He noted how well she treated these girls compared with her attitude toward himself and Will. This reinforced him devaluing his masculinity and valuing femininity. By age five he had become skilled at changing diapers, giving baths, and brushing hair. He also enjoyed joining his younger sisters in playing with dolls. After he had started school, he began tutoring his younger siblings. By the time he was ten, he was preparing breakfast for himself and his siblings. He strived not to be a man, not to be anything really, but just to be his mother's reflection. If there were anything real about him, any edges that stuck out, she would have a target at which to direct her rage. By being her reflection, he could at least get a bit of approval now and then. Meanwhile, he was developing feelings of inferiority about his masculinity and a compensatory attitude of superiority that would form the nucleus of his gender narcissism.

His father, at the same time, was distant. Norbert recalled that when he was four years old his father and older brother went to the World's Fair together. Norbert wanted to go, but his father told him he was too young. He felt excluded from the world of men. At the same time he learned how to manipulate his father as his mother did. He recalled that once, when his father came after him to spank him, he began to shriek hysterically (as he had seen his mother do), and his father laughed and said, "How can I spank you when you shriek like that?" His exclusion from the world of men and his bond with his mother prevented him from resolving his father complex. As he grew older, he found himself admiring his father's chest, and wanting to touch his father while he was sleeping.

While all this was going on, his older brother picked on him mercilessly. Calling Norbert a "goody-two-shoes," a "fairy," and a "queen," Will would pounce on him, pin him to the ground, and force him to say "Uncle" or sometimes "Aunt" or sometimes "You're a wonderful person." These episodes were experienced as rapes. His relationship with his brother also reinforced the development of feelings of masculine inferiority and gender narcissism (a preoccupation with his maleness).

The only place he could go to for solace was art. As a child he had shown talents for all the arts: he excelled at piano, drawing, and literature and was often the star of the elementary school plays. In high school he sang in the chorus, was editor of the yearbook, and appeared in the junior and senior plays. He and his mother sometimes went to New York City (they lived in the suburbs) to see Broadway musicals. Once he wrote and directed a one-act Christmas musical, including five songs, about Jesus and the three wise men. His father, as usual, was busy with his career as a lawyer and his wife didn't bother to tell him about the play. In fact, the only one in his family who attended the performance was his mother. When he asked her afterward how she liked it, she replied, "It was good. But don't get a big head. Let's go. I've got a roast in the oven."

"Until I graduated from high school, it was easy for me to write and direct things—plays, videos, musicals, you name it," Norbert said, lying with his arms stiffly at his sides and his fists clenched, as was his habit. "I never thought twice about it then. Now I think thirty times about everything."

"What happened?" I asked.

"When I was in high school, it didn't have to be professional. Now it does. Now it has to be perfect."

"Perfection is impossible."

"I know. That's why I can't produce anything."

Since Norbert was of the opinion that everything he did had to be perfect, and in order for it to be perfect his body had to be in a state of high tension, he was tense most of the time. He was always ready to fight or flee, always in a state of sympathetic nervous system arousal. He had developed this mode of operation in his family system, where he had had to be ready to cope with the dealings of his family. Now he was convinced he had to maintain this "alertness"—as he called it—to perform at his maximum in his daily adult life. But, in fact, he made many mistakes on his jobs on film crews; moreover, in the areas that were of most concern to him, his stalled movie career and his sexuality, he was at a standstill. He had started several scripts since leaving graduate school but had gotten no further than the first few pages. As for sexuality, until he was twenty-three, he had not even masturbated.

In his early twenties, he had a relationship with a woman. She was the one who took all the initiative in the relationship, and he went along with it. For a while he thought maybe he could be heterosexual, even though he was primarily attracted to men. In his relationship with his girlfriend, he had to be the perfect selfobject for her, as he had been for his mother. Sexually, he had to please her and forget about himself. There could never be any negative thoughts or feelings between them. Everything must be perfect. When it could no longer be that way— when he began having an almost constant undercurrent of negative thoughts about her and impulses toward men—he broke off from her rather than share the negative feelings and thoughts.

His relationships with men were not much better. He was either supercritical of himself or of the men he met. Physically they had to be just right. They had to have a certain kind of chin, certain kind of eyes, certain kind of brows, a certain kind of lips, a certain kind of muscles on their chest, arms, and legs, and especially a certain kind of buttocks. He lusted after a "hunk," who represented to him his ideal of masculinity. This ideal was much like his father as a younger man, about whom he continued to dream. By bonding with such a man, he might dwell in the vitality of his masculinity and become alive and manly. Psychoanalytically, being taken anally by such a "masculine" man might allow for the assuaging of his castration fear and Oedipal guilt, while paving the way for his initiation into the world of men.

As I do with many clients, I worked with Norbert both individually and in a group. One of the advantages of group therapy is that several people give feedback instead of just one. Norbert was in a therapy group of people in the arts, so all of them could empathize with his struggle. In his individual sessions, I pointed out how his smirk and clenched fists served defensive purposes but kept him from becoming real and getting in touch with his feelings. He listened, but didn't really heed. When several people in the group told him they were "turned off" by his smile and pointed out how tense his body language was, he became embarrassed; the group's feedback hit him on a more emotional level.

In group therapy, I'm a bit more eclectic than in individual therapy. The other people provide additional voices and eyes that can be utilized in various exercises. One of the more successful exercises that I did with Norbert was having him role-play various members of his family.

"Talk to your mother. Put her in that empty chair," I said one night.

"I'm really angry at you," he said to the empty chair, the ever-present smirk flickering at the edges of his mouth.

"If you're angry, why are you still smiling?" I asked him.

"Yeah, Norbert, drop the smile," a group member said.

"I don't believe you're really angry," another said.

He tried to get rid of the smirk, but it kept flashing on and off. Clearly, he felt vulnerable without it. "I'm angry at you because you never really saw me," he continued, staring at the empty chair. "I was just your little assistant, just an extension of you. You never knew who I was. I was invisible."

"Now be your mother," I told him. "Sit in the empty chair and be your mother."

He arose, the smirk still on his face, and sat in the other chair. He sat up and spoke in a whiny, self-righteous tone of voice. "Of course I saw you. But I had seven children to take care of and a husband who just sat around drinking beer and watching football." The smirk had gradually faded as he got more into the role. "I had to do everything by myself, cook and clean and do the laundry and go to the PTA meetings. I did the best I could."

"Now be yourself again," I said.

He switched chairs and became more animated. "That's just it. You didn't have to do everything by yourself. You could have had us kids help you, but you didn't. You wanted to be a martyr so that you could complain all the time. I needed love. I needed support. I needed understanding. I hate you for that."

"Good," I said. "Now be your mother again."

He switched chairs, and now his expression became dark and menacing. "How dare you talk to me that way, young man! Who do you think you are? I changed your diapers, and don't you forget that! Don't you *ever* talk to me that way! *Ever,* do you hear! I'll slap you! I'll slap you right across your spoiled little face!" He slapped the air in front of him. He was really getting into the role now. I watched his face carefully and could see that although he was yelling and slapping the air, his eyes were becoming sad. All at once he stopped and sighed and closed his eyes, holding back tears.

"How are you feeling now, Norbert?"

"Hurt, confused. I just had a flashback. I was remembering this time when I was about sixteen, and I was trying to be a little more independent. One day some woman came to our door to ask directions. My mother opened the door and started talking dramatically as she often did, and after a few minutes I said, 'Mom, I think the lady wants to go.' As soon as my mother closed the door, she slapped me and yelled at me for about twenty minutes about what a goddamned brat I was, how I'd better not ever take that attitude with her again."

"Breathe. Let the air out slowly." I was trying to facilitate his letting out his emotions, but like many of us, he had been trained to keep them inside. I enlisted the help of the group.

"While we've got Norbert's mother in the room, does anybody else have anything to say to her?"

"I do," a young male member said. "I'm very angry at you for the way you treated Norbert. I'd like to slap you the way you just slapped him."

"I agree with that," a young woman said. "I hate your guts. You remind me of my own mother. You're so into yourself that you can't see anybody else. Can't you see how hurt your son is? How much he needs your love?"

"I'm very angry at you," another said.

"What does Norbert's mother say?" I asked Norbert. He assumed the role of his mother again, sitting up in the chair with his arms folded. By now there was no longer any smirk at all.

"What do I say? I did the best I could. Sometimes a kid has to be slapped. You wouldn't understand."

"Did *your* mother slap you?" I asked.

"My mother? My mother was a tyrant," Norbert said in a cold, self-righteous tone that apparently mimicked the tone his mother had used in speaking about her own mother. "With my mother you never knew which way the wind was going to blow. If Norbert thinks I'm a bad mother, he should have met his grandmother, may she rest in peace. She didn't just slap; she used to whip us with the branches of trees, and not just on the behind, if you know what I mean."

An exercise like this could go on for the whole hour-and-a-half session of the group. The general aim of the exercise would be to assist Norbert in getting in touch with his feelings. Having him speak to his mother allowed him to explore and vent his own feelings; having him *be* his mother was a way of getting him to see things from her perspective and to permit him to enact his rage at her by exaggerating his portrayal of her. Having the group confront her was helpful because they were able to express anger at her that he himself was unable to do, since he was conflicted between wanting to protect and to condemn her. Hence, they served as a model for him to follow. A by-product of having the group confront his mother was that it demonstrated a kind of support for Norbert's feelings that had been lacking in his childhood and was therefore a reparative experience. Finally, asking the mother about her own childhood and her own mother provided yet another perspective—an empathic recognition that Norbert's mother also had a mother and that each of us in this world has been both child and parent.

Through the combination of analytic work in his individual sessions and exercises such as this one in the group, Norbert gradually resolved his inferiority/superiority conflict and moved forward. He got a job with a major company and was eventually promoted to vice president in charge of film development. His job was to locate properties—movies, plays, and musicals—that could be converted into movie scripts. He would hire a writer to do the screenplay and collaborate with her or him to turn out a script. Then he would hire a director. At some point he intended to do the directing himself. As he became more relaxed, he developed more confidence in his creativity, and the negative voices of his mother and brother diminished.   '

At the same time, his quality of life also began to improve. For a time he dated men, then he went back and dated women again. The conflict between homosexuality and heterosexuality was resolved in favor of the latter, but it didn't come easy. He had great fear that women would turn on him, as he had experienced with his mother. While he worked through these fears, he developed more skills for coping with the rigors of heterosexual dating.

I recognize that controversy exists in the therapeutic community with regard to a therapist helping a patient change his orientation from homosexual or bisexual to heterosexual. Many believe that homosexuals who want to change their orientation, and therapists who assist them, are reacting to—and reinforcing—discrimination against gays. While being sensitive to this point of view, I nevertheless believe that each patient should be perceived on an individual basis. While Norbert had introjected some of society's prejudice against homosexuality, and therefore hated his own gayness, at the same time he was also a religious person who very much wanted a conventional life with a wife and children. For years he volunteered as a mentor, and he really liked children. Hence, his wish to change to a heterosexual orientation was not just an attempt to deny his own gayness, but rather the fulfillment of a deeply felt dream for a certain lifestyle.

Also, when psychodynamic therapy is conducted, people undergo unconscious, automatic change. The working-through process, in which patients talk about past episodes and relationships until they have unraveled the knots that keep them enmeshed in vicious circles in their present lives, has an influence on all aspects of a person's functioning, including sexual functioning. If an individual such as Norbert has been conditioned by a terrifying mother to fear women, and by a cold, distant father to crave bonding with men, the working-through process will gradually diminish such tendencies. Whether research will uncover a genetic predisposition to homosexuality (the Genome Project completed in 2001 didn't find a "gay" gene), one can never discount the environment as a contributing causative factor in sexual orientation. Indeed, the environment is a factor in the varying shades of both heterosexuality and homosexuality—from those who are destructively impulsive to those who are religiously rigid.

Norbert's therapy lasted many years, involving much difficult, detailed work. In movies and plays portraying therapy, one often sees scenes of dramatic breakthroughs; however, in actual therapy, progress is slow and sometimes imperceptible. It is only in retrospect that one becomes aware of the progress made. Sometimes being in therapy is like doing yoga or going to a health club; it's an ongoing pursuit. The process of toning your body or attuning your spirituality never stops, nor does personal growth.

Chapter 8

Priscilla: The Writer
Who Couldn't Hate Her Father

Many people have problems expressing anger, or even acknowledging that they feel it. They view anger as an "evil" emotion and don't want to admit to themselves or others that they harbor such a feeling. However, when anger isn't acknowledged or processed and its origin is not understood, it invariably develops into neurotic defense mechanisms such as denial, projection, displacement, reaction formation, or repression. In the case of artists, unacknowledged anger also translates into blocked creativity. In the case of therapy, it leads to resistance to the treatment and to the therapist.

Priscilla had been seeing me twice a week for nearly a year when the therapy hit an impasse. Each session began in the same manner.

"What should we do today?" she would ask, yawning.

"What would you like to do?"

"I'd like not to be here."

"Where would you like to be?"

"Anywhere but here."

She was an attractive woman of about thirty, quite intelligent and witty in a somewhat caustic way, who had been struggling for many months with unresolved anger toward her parents. She was a writer who could not write, and although she knew her writer's block was somehow connected to her father's ridicule of not only her writing but also her intelligence in general, and to her mother's passivity and deceit (she was silent whenever Priscilla's father mocked her), the anger remained unresolved because it had become transferred onto me.

"Anywhere?" I asked. "That sounds rather vague."

"Outside," she said, gazing out the window at the sunny, summer afternoon. "Outside in the park."

"With me or by yourself?"

"You could come. I wouldn't mind."

"Would we do therapy in the park?"

"No, absolutely not."

"Then what would we do?"

"Whatever we liked."

She gave me a sideways smile. She was caught up in a power struggle with me. I wanted her to do therapy; she wanted to seduce me. It was an angry seductiveness the aim of which was to pull me down from my perch as the "authority figure." This represented a symbolic reenactment of the situation she had endured during her childhood, when she had wanted her father to stop being tyrannical and had tried, in her childlike way, to charm him—without success.

There are parents who, with the best of intentions, nevertheless convey to their children that they lack certain capacities. Such children may then seek to become proficient in the very thing their parents said they lacked. Other parents, due to unconscious competitive feelings toward a child, may go a step further and openly disparage a child's ambitions. Such was the case with Priscilla's father. Apparently, as is often the case, he was repeating with his own daughter a model of relating that he had experienced in his own family. He had had an older sister who, according to Priscilla, had teased him and belittled him, with the result that he had always felt inferior to her. Now, with his own daughter, he seemed to have transferred this sibling relationship onto his daughter, in reverse. Unwittingly, he had assumed a mocking tone toward his own daughter's intellectual pursuits.

One telling memory that Priscilla related was of her writing and illustrating a children's book when she was six years old. She purposely worked on the book while her father was in the room, seated on the rug beneath the chair where he always read his newspaper, hoping he would notice. When he didn't, she sidled up to him, pressing her belly against his big arm, and smiling her sweetest smile as she held out her book. He quickly glanced through it, handed it back to her, and replied, "You misspelled three words, and a cow doesn't look like that." When she showed it to her mother, the latter sat down with her and read the whole book, praising her efforts. "That's beautiful." But she didn't put much stock in her mother's words, for her mother tended to like everything she did. It was her critical father whom she desperately wanted to please. She ran back to her father to tell him, "Mommy likes my book."

"That's good," he replied without looking up.

Later, she cried in her mother's lap, "I hate my daddy! I hate him, I hate him." Being a passive woman, dependent on her husband's approval, she couldn't really validate Priscilla's feelings. Instead, she defended her husband, saying, "Don't talk like that. Your father's a little eccentric, but he means well and he really loves you. You should never be angry at your father." Her mother was never angry at her father or at anybody, and Priscilla learned to handle her anger the same way—that is, to deny it.

Priscilla seemed to have an Electra complex with all the usual fantasies of taking her mother's place in the master bedroom. But her childhood attempts at seduction ended in frustration. On one occasion, at around the same age, Priscilla had asked her father to run away with her and marry her. He had promised her he would, and they had made plans. However, later he had brought it up in front of his wife and joked about it. "Priscilla and I are going to run off and get married!"

"Oh really?" the mother had beamed.

"Not!" the father added caustically.

"That was a secret," Priscilla shot in.

"Sorry."

She continued to write and draw without conflict until her college years. But during her senior year something happened that changed Priscilla's life. I had no doubts that she was talented. In college she had placed first in a fiction-writing contest, and upon graduation she had had several stories accepted by literary quarterlies. I had read some of her writing and found it delightful; she had an ear for ironic dialogue. However, she had made the mistake of sending a copy of a quarterly containing one of her stories to her parents. Her father never acknowledged receiving it. Her interest in writing began to wane.

Her therapy hit an impasse as more and more anger at her parents began to surface. It seemed as if the more memories she had about her parents, the more seductive she became toward me. The more I wanted her to talk about her parents and work through the feelings, the more she wanted to talk about me and get me to abandon my role as therapist. If I asked her to talk about her father, she'd ask me to talk about mine. If I asked her to talk about her mother, she'd want to talk about mine. If I asked her about her dreams, she'd want to know what I dreamed about and if I ever dreamed about patients. If I gave her a writing assignment (to help loosen up her writer's block), suggesting that she write about something about her childhood, she'd come back with a page about my supposed childhood. If I did a Gestalt exercise with her, asking her to imagine that her father or mother were sitting in an empty chair, she'd say, "That's silly. Why should I talk to an empty chair? Why don't we go out and have coffee instead?"

Meanwhile, as more and more of this anger got transferred onto me, Priscilla's life outside the therapy office had become increasingly problematic. She had been having serious fights with her husband, and she had a series of "accidents," the most recent of which involved a bicycle crash that left her sprained and bruised and hospitalized. The day after she got out of the hospital, she called me to ask if I made house calls.

"It's my policy not to make house calls," I explained. In fact, I had no such policy, but I knew that under the circumstances it would be inappropriate. "I'll do a telephone session with you, though."

"No, that's all right," she snapped. "I'll just have to wait until I'm able to come to the office. I don't know when that will be."

My refusal to make a house call brought on the impasse. Was it the right thing to do? I questioned myself about that, and recalled case histories from the literature in which therapists had worked differently with patients. Some therapists have even taken patients into their homes to live for a while (Winnicott, 1947; Rosen, 1962), reasoning that by joining a patient's resistance, they would "soften" the patient and convince him or her to give it up. Freud noted in his paper "Observations on Transference-Love" (1915) that the erotic transference was one of the most difficult to resolve, since it was both an act of sexuality and of aggression. He advised preserving it for purposes of analysis, while neither discouraging nor gratifying it. However, he added that there were some women with whom this policy would not work: "These are women of an elemental passionateness; they tolerate no surrogates; they are children of nature who refuse to accept the spiritual instead of the material." With such women the therapist was forced to make a choice "either to return their love or else bring down upon oneself the full force of the mortified woman's fury" (p. 386). Another line of therapeutic thinking, one advocated by Kernberg, Selzer, and Koenigsberg (1989), seeks to force the patient's aggression to the surface by setting firm boundaries. This is the approach I followed by refusing to make the house visit.

When she returned to therapy, a week later, she was aloof, moody, and more caustic than usual. The message was, if I would not give her what she wanted, she would not give me what I wanted. Whereas before she had at least pretended to listen to interpretations, now she simply turned away and yawned. Her sessions were full of silences, yawns, and complaints about boredom. Several weeks passed in this vein.

She was still acting out her anger, so I had to try another technique. Sometimes, in treating people in the arts, art therapy interventions are effective. She had shown a talent for drawing at an early age, and I reasoned that, if I used art as a vehicle to get to her underlying conflicts, she would not be as defensive as she was when I tried using verbal technique, since her strongest defense seemed to be the intellectual defense of using words to mock me (as her father had done to her). Anyway, she had been complaining about being bored with the usual routine and talking about doing some kind of art that would represent a breaking of the routine.

When I got out the colored pencils and drawing pad, a smile crept onto her mouth. She was clearly bemused, if still angry. "You want me to draw pictures? Why not? Do you think it will cure me?" She shot me a crooked grin.

"I think it might provide us with some insights."

"Oh, good. I love insights."

She sat on the rug to do the drawings while I remained in my chair, observing. She did the drawings in an offhanded manner, smiling all the while as though it were a joke. I asked her to draw a house, a tree, and a person. Instead of a house, she drew a lighthouse. Instead of a tree, she drew a telephone pole. Instead of a person, she drew a person (girl) standing under a tree. When she had finished, I picked up the last drawing, the girl standing under a tree, and studied it. Her penciling was light, the tree and person were very small, and there was a considerable amount of white space. The white space, I knew, was indicative of hostility—hostility toward her childhood (she had drawn a little girl)—and perhaps also to the therapy office.

"Well," she said, "what do you think, doctor? How sick am I?"

"Do you really want to hear my interpretation, or is that a rhetorical question?"

"Sure. Let's hear it. Do I have a choice?"

"Of course you have a choice. You always have a choice."

"All right. I'm game." She smiled suspiciously.

"Are you sure?"

"I'm sure."

I tried the first interpretation, observing Priscilla carefully. "You see all this white space? You see how small you made this drawing, and how lightly you penciled it? That usually indicates withdrawal, lack of commitment, and repressed anger."

"I know all that. It's true. I'm not committed. I don't have any friends. I've withdrawn from everybody, including my husband. So? What else is new?"

"We don't have to do this if you don't want to."

"No, no. Go on. Tell me more about the drawings, so I can be enlightened and mature."

I was aware of her sarcasm, but I also sensed that the sarcasm was a bit less rigid than usual. Pointing to the clouds hovering over the roof of the lighthouse she had drawn, I asked, "What do these clouds mean to you?"

"I would suppose you want me to say it's depression."

"And what do you think it means that the lighthouse you've drawn is leaning as if it's about to fall?"

"I guess maybe it's fragile. Maybe it's about to fall. Maybe I'm about to fall?" She smiled at me with all her teeth.

"And what about this tree? It's not a tree at all. It's a telephone pole. What does that mean?"

"Maybe that I want to make a telephone call."

"Right. Very funny. But what does it mean that it has no branches and no leaves?"

"Like you said, I'm not committed. I'm not reaching out."

"And what about this little girl here? Why do you think you drew a little girl?"

"Maybe I feel like a little girl."

"And why is the little girl sitting with her arms folded and her head down."

"I don't know. Why don't *you* tell *me*? You're the doctor."

"Perhaps she's sad and angry."

"Very interesting. But what does it prove? I know all that already."

I put the drawings down and studied her. She stood up and sat back down in her chair, facing me. I sensed she was angry about the interpretations but, as usual, was not expressing this anger directly. "How do you feel about our interpretations?"

"They give me something to think about. Yes, I'll think about them. Is that what I'm supposed to do?"

She was always asking me what she was supposed to do. "No," I answered. "That's not what you're supposed to do. But if you want to think about them, you may."

"Thank you, doctor. I'll think about them then."

Priscilla did not mention the drawings during the next session, nor the one after that, nor the one after that. Once again the impasse had seemingly settled in, and now the silence with regard to her response to the drawings became a part of the impasse. I did not wish to bring up the subject first, as she had a tendency to feel coerced by me whenever I initiated anything. The summer days seemed to linger, along with the impasse. Finally, after a month, at the beginning of the session, she brought it up.

"What shall we do today?"

"What would you like to do?"

"I knew you were going to ask that. Well, we could do another drawing."

"We could. Why do you want to do another drawing?"

"You seemed to get so much out of the last ones I did."

"Oh? How so?"

"The exercise made you feel so powerful. You could sit back and analyze me. Point out my faults."

"So, you think I got some pleasure out of interpreting your drawings?"

"Of course. People always get pleasure out of finding fault in other people."

"Who gets pleasure out of finding your faults?"

"You want me to say 'my father,' right?"

"Did he do that?"

"Oh, yes. Constantly." She looked up at me as though slightly shocked by this admission. "I don't want to talk about my father."

"All right. Let's not talk about him."

"Let's talk about the drawings."

"All right."

"Shall we look at the drawings again?"

"All right."

I opened the drawer where I kept the drawings and took them out. She sat in her chair, watching me with a slight smirk.

"Would you stop being so agreeable?" she said.

"How would you like me to be?"

"I'd like you to be angry at me."

"What would that do for you?"

"Then . . . then I could also be angry at you without feeling guilty."

"Yes, and then maybe you could also feel angry at your father without feeling guilty."

"Shut up about my father."

"All right."

"My father has nothing to do with this!" Priscilla glared at me and her eyes became sad and dark. "Why do you keep bringing up my father? You're doing that just to annoy me, aren't you? I don't want to be depressed and angry. I don't want to be sad. I don't want to hate my father . . ."

"I know."

"And I don't want to . . . cry . . ."

"I know."

She broke into sobs, huddled in her chair like a small, lonesome child. The summer sun swept brightly into the room, and she shielded her eyes from it and from me with a self-conscious forearm, as I looked silently and gratefully on.

Chapter 9

Alex: The Painter
Who Was Too Refined
to Be Commercial

One of the most controversial contributions of Spotnitz to the psychoanalytic literature is the concept of the toxoid response, an extension of Winnicott's notion of the therapeutic use of objective hate (1947), Reich's character analysis (1933), and Jacobson's timed expression of anger (1971). In his classic paper, "The Toxoid Response," Spotnitz writes that "in cases of schizophrenia, psychotic depression and other severe disturbances, one encounters resistances, chiefly preverbal, that do not respond to objective interpretation. Their resolution is thwarted by toxic affects that have interfered with the patient's maturation and functioning" (Spotnitz, 1976, p. 49). He compares this to the situation of a person who has a virus and does not respond to warmth, rest, and diet, but must be injected with a mild case of that virus itself so that he or she develops antibodies and becomes immunized against it. Likewise, according to Spotnitz, in treating patients who have been infected with an "emotional virus," the psychoanalyst must "inject" them with a mild case of that virus in order to help them develop the emotional antibodies needed to immunize themselves against it.

When a narcissistic patient begins acting out rage toward the analyst, the analyst develops a narcissistic countertransference—becoming infected with the patient's feelings. The analyst, according to Spotnitz, must then conduct a self-analysis to ensure that the rage has been induced entirely by the patient (objective countertransference) and not by his or her own unresolved psychopathology (subjective countertransference). If it is determined that the rage has been induced by the patient, the analyst may decide to administer a dose of this rage back to the patient. The patient "is given verbal injections of the emotions he has induced in the analyst, carefully 'treated' to destroy their toxicity and to stimulate the formation of antibodies," Spotnitz explains. "In brief, the induced emotions are employed as a toxoid" (1976, p. 50). Spotnitz cautions that this intervention is not to be used indiscriminately, for it can cause damage to the patient if the therapist is not sure that his countertransference is objective.

In his case history about Fred, Spotnitz demonstrated the use of the toxoid response. At a certain point in the therapy, Fred began making threats about wanting to get off the couch to attack Spotnitz. He would make these threats and then lapse into silence. Spotnitz encouraged Fred to continue to verbalize his anger, but Fred resisted. "Feelings of guilt about what he might say clammed him up. He also had strong fears that talking about his impulses would force him to act on them. He was convinced that his destructive urges proved that he was incurable" (p. 54). Nevertheless, Fred's threats continued and Spotnitz noticed that they were arousing a great deal of resentment in him. When Fred boasted of the uniqueness of his capacity for violence, Spotnitz became even more resentful. That's when he decided to give Fred a toxoid response. The next time Fred threatened him, Spotnitz threatened him back. However, his response was too mild and did not match Fred's ferocity, which prompted Fred to reply, "Don't try that stuff. You're repeating what I say, but you don't feel it" (p. 55). Spotnitz understood that Fred needed more than mimicry; he needed a mirror image. Spotnitz bided his time, allowing the induced rage to build up inside him. A few sessions later, Fred exploded during the middle of the session, "I'll bash your head in." "No you won't," Spotnitz exploded back with equal rage, "because I'll bash yours in before you can get off the couch" (p. 55).

Fred was awed, Spotnitz reports, by this outburst and exclaimed that Spotnitz really did hate him as much as he hated Spotnitz and could be even more vicious. Hence, Fred garnered relief and security from the carefully treated toxiod response of Spotnitz. Repeated responses of this sort helped to immunize Fred and give him the antibodies he needed to fight against the emotional toxicity within himself and from the outside world. He became less terrified of his destructive urges, and they gradually lost their toxic quality. He saw that somebody he respected could accept and verbalize such urges in a constructive way and learned to do so himself.

Spotnitz and other modern psychoanalysts (Epstein and Feiner, 1979; Marshall, 1979; Meadow, 1987; Margolis, 1987) have put an emphasis on providing detailed descriptions of and rationales for the use of emotional communication and the toxoid response in treatment. However, it is also important to have a theoretical base for the understanding of how patients are infected with the "emotional viruses" that underlie their narcissism and later require a toxoid response as a remedy. Spotnitz (1985) only vaguely refers to a process in which individuals become "defective" to the degree that their maturational needs are not met in their interchanges with "natural objects" during their childhoods, particularly during the first two years of life. He then notes that such maturational failures induce a rage reaction in children which must be suppressed in order to protect their parents. Narcissistic children (particularly those who suffer from severe forms of depression or schizophrenia) then withdraw into a shell, protecting primary objects and themselves from this rage while they erect an illusory world in which they are in some way powerful in order to compensate for their inner feelings of powerlessness.

Experimental psychology provides a more explicit theory of this developmental process. Seligman (1992) demonstrated through experiments with dogs that animals can be programmed to be helpless. In his experiment, two groups of mongrel dogs were given repeated shocks. One group could stop the shocks by pushing a lever. The other group had no lever to push and couldn't stop the shocks. Without any way of stopping them, the second group of dogs soon stopped trying to do anything at all, simply stood there apathetically accepting the shocks (similar to what happens when one is depressed). Later, when this second group was put in another cage in which it was given ways to escape the shocks, 80 percent of the group accepted the shocks without even trying to escape. Seligman termed this "learned helplessness" and linked it with depression.

In treating a number of artists with narcissistic personalities, some of whom have suffered from this sense of helplessness along with the associated narcissism and rage, I have come to understand what I believe is a common form of pathogenic object relationship, one that contributes significantly to bringing about the formation of a narcissistic personality and a narcissistic defense structure. The understanding of how the narcissistic personality is formed helps to explain why emotional communication such as the toxoid response is necessary in its treatment.

Based on my observations, the essence of the development of narcissism is that children become infected through contact with caretakers who themselves are infected. It is a process in which narcissistic caretakers will affirm their false, grandiose selves by enlisting their children as selfobjects. Such caretakers are invariably abusive emotionally, sexually, or physically, but deny such abuse. So their children must learn to also deny the abuse, and they develop the defense mechanism of splitting. In the previous chapters of this book, I have recounted several examples of this kind of parent-child interaction. Certainly Norbert's mother, who needed him to affirm that she was the perfect mother despite her constant attacks on his masculinity, fell into this category, as well as Priscilla's father, who demanded to be idealized by his daughter and wife while denying that his mocking attitude toward Priscilla was abusive.

During the process of parent-child interaction an accumulation of rage builds up inside the children. Over the years they attempt to verbalize their rage, but their narcissistic caretakers make them feel guilty and shameful when they do so. Eventually they learn not only to withhold their rage, but also to doubt their perceptions of reality. When these children become adults they relate to others in a manner similar to the way caretakers related to them as children. To use the terminology of Spotnitz, they have become infected with emotional toxins, and they then unconsciously infect those around them. Schematically, this process can be outlined as follows:

1. Caretaker demands perfect attunement or conduct from child.
2. Caretaker attacks child with doses of rage when perfection is not attained.
3. Caretaker thwarts all attempts at counter-rage by child.
4. Caretaker denies, disowns, or projects the enraged part of his or her self.
5. Caretaker shames child when child tries to point out reality, adding insult to injury, hence child's perceptions become confused.
6. Child develops narcissistic character, depression, and delusional grandiosity; as an adult he or she repeats and reverses what was done in childhood.

I didn't use the toxoid response with Alex until the last moment. Alex saw himself as a sensitive, refined intellectual, an artist and man of the world, a superior and elite person, and I mirrored that view. In actuality, he did possess many of these qualities and gifts, but nearly all had remained fairly undeveloped. Since college, he had hardly been able to produce any new art; he worked at menial jobs such as waitering and often got fired from such jobs; he was deeply in debt; he had no male friends and had never maintained a lasting relationship with a woman. He managed to sustain his delusion of superiority through a repetitive pattern in which he enlisted others—mainly women—into becoming selfobjects, which he then became bored with (because of their "inferiority") and dumped (injected with his rage). He never viewed himself as an angry or rageful person, however, and prided himself on how sensitively he let the women down, usually after extracting much in the way of financial help from them.

He fit the description of a schizoid personality: he was withdrawn and defended against attachment through talk. From the beginning of his treatment, Alex filled the room with talk. "Do you think artists are messengers of sorts?" he would ask, resting on my couch, his arms behind his head, and then continuing without a pause. "I had a mentor in college who used to say that all the time. I used to think he was being a bit presumptuous, but now I dare say he may have been right. As Shelley put it, 'Truth and beauty is all you need to know.' Or was it Keats? I always get those two mixed up." He could talk for sessions without wanting any feedback from me. He talked of his art, his philosophy, his exploits with women, basking in our relationship. He had formed a twinship transference with me; I was an idealized figure, a psychoanalyst (a profession he admired), and he was the artist-savant who was on a plane with me, who understood things almost as well as I did (perhaps better in some ways). Yet, despite this seemingly idealized view of me, I was relegated to an extremely limited role; I was there only to mirror and join him, only to agree with his every utterance and support his every decision, or to remain silent if I could not.

Even agreeing with Alex was tricky. For instance, sometimes I would simply repeat to him a key word in the form of a question. He might say, "I have problems relating with women," then hesitate for just a moment, almost as if to bait me. "Problems?" I would ask. He would then reply, "Well, not really problems. I relate to them well, actually." For the next fifteen or twenty minutes, sometimes until the end of the session, he would defend his record with women. I soon found that the only safe thing to do was to simply say, "I see," or "That's interesting."

It was impossible for me to engage him in any way. If I tried to engage him, he would divert the conversation into an endless monologue that served to keep me at a distance. Even basic interactions between us had to be handled gingerly. When I asked him at the end of a session if he could have his check written out in advance, he became so offended that a week or so later he wanted to quit therapy. The reason he gave for wanting to leave therapy—not being able to afford it—had nothing to do with this incident. I had to remind him that I had asked him to have his checks written out in advance the week before, and even though he finally admitted to being a little bothered by the incident, he nevertheless denied its relevance to his wanting to leave.

During the course of his ramblings, he described his pattern with women in great detail. He would meet a new woman and quickly seduce her—usually the same night he met her. He would present himself as a sensitive, intelligent artist who knew how to treat a woman. Soon she was living with him, then lending him money. At the point when she began talking about marriage, he would become critical of her. She was not sophisticated enough, not beautiful enough, not confident enough. He would constantly correct her grammar, review her apparel, remind her that she was watching television too much (and low-brow shows at that), and pick up after her. Soon arguments occurred, which became more and more protracted. Then either he would inform her that the relationship was not working out and they would have to separate, or she would get the message and leave. Never was there any desire on his part to try to discuss and resolve problems at this point. I perceived a great deal of passive aggression in this pattern. Yet, I couldn't say anything.

Just as it was easy for Alex to seduce new women, it was also easy for him to get new jobs, but not easy for him to keep them. He could walk into a fairly nice restaurant, ask to see the manager, and quickly convince the manager that his knowledge of wines was extraordinary, his manners impeccable, and his restaurant skills were well rounded. He would be hired and put into some special situation; even though he might be a trainee, the manager or head waiter would consult with him about the wine or other operations. However, before very long he would begin acting like a prima donna, and soon the manager, other employees, and even customers were demanding his ouster. Yet, no matter how many jobs he lost, he would somehow not really examine his own contribution to the firing. He would conclude that the manager, if a woman, was a "man hater" (or, if it were a man, he was jealous of his knowledge, his intellect, his attractiveness to women); he would castigate fellow employees for their mercenary tactics, implying that his only failing was that he refused to sell his soul to the restaurant; and in general he would complain that he was a pearl among swine. Again, as he reported these events, I could not say a word.

Despite his talk about art, his production of paintings was minimal and the works he produced were seemingly designed to have mini-mal impact on the viewer. Every year or so he would manage to convince the restaurant at which he was working to allow him to exhibit his work on the premises. These weren't fine restaurants, but rather Soho or Greenwich Village cafés, and the customers tended to be strung-out college students who couldn't afford to buy paintings. Whenever he had these shows, he would hurriedly knock out a few new works to go along with his old ones. I had the impression that what was important was not the art itself but the fact of having a show now and then to prove that he was actually a working artist.

In my estimation he did have talent, but that talent was quite latent. The paintings he succeeded in eking out were abstracts done in pastels or watercolors. Sometimes the lines and colors were so faint one could hardly see them. They were the kinds of paintings one might use for décor, the same way one might put up a pretty but unobtrusive curtain. My interpretation of his work was that it served an unconscious pur-pose. Just as he maintained his narcissistic distance with people, so too he kept figures and meaningful compositions out of his paintings; there were only patterns and designs, denoting his narcissistic isolation from people and his splitting off of his own real self. His paintings were intel-lectual exercises, just as were most of his early sessions with me.

When I asked Alex why he didn't try to get his work in galleries, he replied that it was because he was always busy struggling to find new jobs or to fix up new lofts that he had gone into debt buying. But mainly he said he did not approach galleries because he regarded the art mar-ketplace as beneath him, a den of gross commercialism that would de-vour his soul. "As my mentor in college used to put it, the New York art scene is a haven for lost souls. I don't really care how much money I make from my paintings. Indeed, I'd rather not make much money. If I did, I'd be enslaved by it and lose all self-respect." He did not go to any showings or cultivate any friendships with fellow artists because other artists had "gone commercial." This left him isolated and depressed.

Perhaps it has become apparent by now that Alex aroused feelings of annoyance. I found myself annoyed at him often—as I did, for example, when he rambled on and didn't let me in, or when he described his pattern of exploiting and then dumping girlfriends. Fortunately, he filled me in on his childhood and as I understood why he was the way he was, I was able to put my annoyance aside and empathize with him.

It became clear that Alex's dysfunctional family had given him toxic responses to his early infantile needs, and that he had devised a narcissistic defensive mode to deal with it. His history is full of abandonment and deception.

His parents married two weeks after they met, and his mother gave birth to Alex scarcely nine months later. A month after that his mother was pregnant with her second child, a girl. A year into the marriage, his father took off, never to be seen again. Hence, Alex grew up without any memory of his father. Nor did he even know what the man looked like, since his mother had thrown away all his pictures, even those in which he posed with his two children.

It seems likely that the period following his father's departure must have been traumatic. Alex was only a month old. In view of what he reported about his mother's relationship to him later, Alex and I speculated that she must have been rejecting him even at that time. She felt betrayed and abandoned by her husband and probably displaced her feelings about him onto her children, particularly her son. He was named after his father and had become, in the mother's mind, symbolic of him.

How did she hold him when she was nursing him? How did she look at him? Did she look at him lovingly, or with a depressed glare? Did she hold him tightly, or did she hold him grudgingly? When he cried, did she go to him or did she let him cry while she lay in bed brooding? Of course we cannot know any of this, we can only theorize that due to the abrupt breakup of her marriage, his mother could not respond appropriately to his infantile needs. From our knowledge of how things usually go in such circumstances, and from the information about how his mother treated him later, such conjecture would probably be appropriate. Apparently a major oral fixation resulted from this early rift and its consequences. The fact that his mother never talked about his father or encouraged her children to do so meant that they never had a chance to mourn his loss and that their perceptions were not affirmed. In other words, Alex was conditioned from birth on not to deal with feelings. The absence of his father was in itself a symbolic form of evading and avoiding; and this is exactly the mode of behavior that became prominent in Alex's life.

Instead of being adored by his mother, he was only marginally wanted. Instead of being a delight, he was a burden. Two of his earliest memories indicate the nature of her attitude toward him. In the first, when he was about four, he was sitting in the kitchen with his aunt and mother. His aunt had not had any children and wondered what it would be like to nurse. With his mother's approval, she took the four-year-old boy and put him at her breast. Alexander felt a mixture of pleasure and humiliation. When he was about five, he ran into the house with a gash on his forehead, having fallen in the snow. When his mother saw his crying, bloody face, she laughed. Only after he had cried out in agony for several minutes did she take him into the bathroom and treat his wound. When he continued to cry, she told him to stop being such a baby.

These two memories are indications of her own degree of narcissism: her self-centeredness, her inability to be empathic toward her son, her lack of respect for his needs and feelings. In the first, she allowed her sister to inappropriately breast-feed a four-year-old, disregarding the consequences of such an action. In the second, she laughed at the boy's injury rather than showing concern, and then compounded this injury by telling him that his feelings about and perceptions of what had happened were wrong ("stop being a baby").

"I never felt that my mother accepted me or knew me," he told me one day. "Indeed, she never accepted or knew anybody. Almost every year she had a relationship with a different man. Almost every year the family would move to a different town. Almost every year I went to a different school. It was dizzying." In each relationship, his mother would fall in love with a man and shortly after would lose interest. No man was ever good enough for her. Her breakups would be sudden and sometimes ugly, and once, one of her ex-lovers set fire to their trailer.

After he had been in therapy with me for a few years, Alex began to seek out information about his father. He called his aunts and uncles, town officials, teachers. Finally he located his father's second wife, and she told him a story about his parents' breakup that differed greatly from his mother's sketchy version. In this version, his father had left his mother because when he had been away from home (he was a salesman), she had had an affair. When Alex confronted his mother about this new story, his mother chastised him for "going behind my back" to talk to the "home wrecker who took my husband away from me."

Alex did not know what to believe, but it was clear that his childhood had been filled with deception on both sides. In addition, a clearer picture of his father now emerged of an impulsive and passive man who had married and divorced a series of women, unable to commit to any of them. This raised the question of whether this mode of relating to women was in part a biological predisposition, since Alex had never known his father and could not have modeled himself after him. He also learned from his father's second wife that his father had not visited him because she hadn't wanted him to. Hence, Alex senior's conduct seemed to hinge partly on his subservience to his second wife.

Later in the analysis, Alex gradually realized his anger at his mother. Since he had never known his father, it was easier to channel all his anger at his mother. What particularly angered him during this period were the memories of the presents she gave him at Christmas and on his birthday. She never got him what he asked for. If he asked for a certain make of bicycle, she would end up getting him a cheaper model. If he asked for flannel shirts, she would get him knitted shirts. If he wanted a game, she would get him a shirt, saying he was too old for games. Her disregard for what he wanted became symbolic in his mind of her lack of respect for his feelings. After a year of investigating his father, he wrote his mother two long letters in which he addressed all the things that had hurt him over the years. She ignored the first letter, and responded to the second with a short note that evaded everything he had said and dismissed it with the sentence, "I did read your letter and realized that you were still being Alex. I do very much hope you get over this soon."

The more I learned about his childhood, the more evident it became that in the transference, as in all other relationships, Alex was copying what was done to him by his parents. Just as his mother kept everybody away, including Alex, so Alex now kept everyone away, including me. Just as his mother quietly hated men (while pretending to love them), so Alex quietly hated women (while pretending to love them). Just as his mother passive-aggressively infected Alex and all others with her narcissistic rage, so Alex passive-aggressively infected the women in his life, his employers, and eventually me, with that same rage.

During the course of his therapy, he had many ways of acting out the rage. One of the most prominent was to ask for my feedback. Then when I started to give it to him, he would interrupt me and defend himself for the rest of the session. If I tried to point out what he had just done, he would say, "I see what you mean," and then defend that for the rest of the session. I learned that it was best to answer all his questions with questions.

After seven years, he came in and said he had made a decision, and he was afraid his decision was going to upset me. As soon as he said this, I knew he had decided to quit therapy, and I was upset. His reasons were the standard ones. He couldn't afford it, and he wanted to see if he could do without therapy. He had recently been fired from another job—that was true. He had also rented a huge loft, which had overextended him financially, and he plunged further into debt. He had just broken up with his latest girlfriend, so she was moving out, and he would have to pay the full rent.

I realized that Alex was acting out transference feelings, and I knew why he was doing it. When he had begun having difficulty with his latest girlfriend, he had asked for my advice. Usually I did not give advice, even upon request, but since this was an emergency I had suggested that he seek couples therapy. A few weeks later he told me his girlfriend had decided to move out, and he was relieved. He made no mention of couples therapy, and I knew he had rejected the idea. He didn't ask for any feedback, and I knew he didn't want any. He had criticized his girlfriend and degraded her until she could tolerate it no more. In short, he had driven her out of the relationship. She was a young woman, twenty years his junior, who wanted to marry him and bear his child. He spoke quite calmly about their separation, feeling nothing. I was experiencing his feelings for him: rage. He was displacing the rage toward his mother onto his latest girlfriend by summarily dumping her.

I had found myself once again feeling annoyed at him over the way he had exploited and dumped this latest girlfriend. This annoyance (countertransference) had caused me to rush in and offer advice that I knew, deep down, he would not receive. To him, this advice meant I was on his girlfriend's side. If I was not perfectly aligned with him, then I was his enemy. Therefore, like her, I had to be dumped.

However, I was ready for this maneuver, for he had done it before, many times, and I had prepared a reply. By abruptly quitting in this "innocent" way, he was recreating the agression and denial of his mother toward him. He had injected me with a toxin. I waited until he had lapsed into a silence, and then I gave him a toxoid response.

"Actually, I have *also* been thinking about terminating the therapy," I said, with just a bit of anger in my voice. In order to mirror him properly, I had to have just about the same amount of anger in my voice as he had in his.

"You have?" He looked around from the couch to study my eyes, wanting to see if I meant it. I actually did. I had to really mean it so that the intervention would have the proper effect.

"Yes, and I was also afraid to tell you because I thought *you* might get upset," I added. "Should we end it right now?"

"*You* sound upset."

"Yes, I am a little annoyed."

"That's interesting." I could see he was quite stunned. For perhaps the first time, I wasn't being a selfobject. Instead of telling him what he wanted to hear, I was telling him what he needed to hear. I was being a real person very much like himself. "Why do you want to terminate the therapy?" he asked in a confused voice.

"I haven't been getting the cooperation from you that I need in order to help you resolve your blocks. That has frustrated me."

"Oh? That's a surprise to me. How have I not been cooperating?"

I proceeded to tell him how he hadn't been cooperating with me from the beginning and tied it to a somewhat lengthy interpretation about his childhood, the loss of his father, and the ambivalence toward this father that was evident in his relationship with me. I also brought in his relationships with women, including the girlfriend he had just rejected, and drew a parallel between his relations with women and his mother's relations with men. Finally I noted that his reluctance to market his paintings was a fear of competition, and I traced this to his lack of a father figure who could have taught him to compete. For the first time in years of therapy, he seemed to listen.

"You're really angry with me, aren't you?" he said.

"Yes, I am. And you're angry with me too!"

"I guess I am."

This response served its purpose. It prodded him out of his defensive posture and aroused first anger and then curiosity. I had given him back a dose of his own medicine, administered at just the right time. Hence, he had been made to acknowledge his anger at me and how he was acting it out. Spotnitz, in his case history about Fred, asserted that Fred garnered relief and security from Spotnitz's emotional response to him. Likewise, I believe Alex felt relieved and secure after my response. When individuals continually act out passive-aggressively toward other persons, even though they may deny the aggression, they nevertheless unconsciously know about it and feel guilty about it. The normal response to passive-aggression is not to acknowledge it—since the perpetrator isn't doing so. The aggression ends up floating around the room like an invisible cloud, making both people tense. When Alex's aggression was reciprocated, the tension dissipated. I had met the test. He had been looking for a father figure who would be strong enough to lead him out of the wilderness in which he was lost. When I showed him that I, too, could be angry and that it was all right with me that I was angry, he felt more secure about me and was more willing to take responsibility for his own anger. When I demonstrated to him that I could compete on his level of acting out, he understood something about friendly competition and mutual respect, something he had never learned from his own father.

Alex ended up staying in therapy for several more years. Our relationship gradually became more authentic, and as it did, the rest of his life, including his art, began to change. He ventured out of the "safety" of pastels and watercolors and into the more challenging world of oil paintings. Before long, he had met a female gallery owner who admired his new work and offered him first a group show and then a solo show.

"So do you feel you've sold out?" I asked him when he told me about the solo show.

"I hope I sell out," he replied with a smirk. "I hope I sell every painting in the show! Wouldn't that be great?"

Chapter 10

Marvin: The Perverse Playwright

When Marvin entered treatment he had stopped writing and directing plays entirely; indeed, he had not written a play since he had graduated from college seven years earlier. In college he had written, directed, and acted in a number of one-act musicals for an experimental acting group he and some friends had formed, but in the intervening years he had not been able to sit down at his computer and write. I had seen many clients who had told similar stories: It's certainly easier to produce creative work in college, when it is either required or supported by the collegial atmosphere than it is afterward, when one must be a self-starter. However, I wanted to get his take on it, so I asked him why he thought he had stopped.

"God only knows! I was hoping you could tell me that," he said in his buoyant manner, chuckling ebulliently. In the early days of his treatment, I always had the feeling that he was performing, trying with all his might to be the best therapy client who ever walked through my door. "I know, I know, I'm supposed to just say whatever comes into my head. Why aren't I writing and directing plays? Why? Why? Why? Because you're an idiot! Don't mind me, I always talk to myself. Anyway, I'm sure you're looking for something a little deeper than that. Why? Why? Why? Well, what comes to mind is that I don't feel good enough to write or direct a play. I mean, I could direct a play if I had to, but I'd be self-conscious the whole time, wondering when the cast and crew would figure out that I'm an idiot."

He was about thirty when he started therapy, but he looked much younger. He had the appearance of a pudgy adolescent, with his T-shirt, jeans, and red, high-top sneakers. Lying in front of me on my couch, I could see his rosy cheeks and his round belly wobbling as he chuckled, and he chuckled a lot.

"What do you mean when you call yourself an idiot?" I said to him in a tone of curiosity. "Can you expand on that?"

"Can I expand on it? Probably not," he chuckled. "But I will. Let's see. Expand, expand, expand. I'm trying, but nothing's coming. Think, idiot, think."

"Let me put it a different way. What thoughts come to you when you write or direct?"

"I don't have any thoughts," he said, chuckling again. "Well, no. That's not true. Whenever I write I think nobody's going to want to read it because they'll see that I'm an idiot. And if I direct, they'll also see that I'm an idiot, only they'll see it more quickly. And God knows what would happen if I tried to act. Then it would really be obvious."

"But what does the word 'idiot' mean to you?"

"What does it mean? I'm sorry; I'm blocking. Oh, God. Have you ever had a patient like me?"

"Finish this sentence: 'I'm an idiot because I' . . . "

"I'm an idiot because . . . I'm an idiot. I'm sorry, I know I'm not helping. I'm an idiot because . . . I'm stupid. No, no, no. Think! All right. I can do this. I'm an idiot because . . . I can't do this simple word association test! I don't know. Are you looking for a particular answer?"

His reaction to this exercise was an example of one of his major problems: Marvin was always pressing, always trying too hard to do things perfectly and then failing at them. He was always trying too hard at jobs, too hard at relationships, and too hard at writing and directing. Always, a voice in his head told him how stupid he was (his superego, in psychoanalytic terms) and this voice was so harsh and so constant he could seldom escape it. The only way he escaped it was by rebelling against it through perverse thinking and behavior. In other words, he had a weak ego, and, therefore, he was caught up in a continual conflict between his harsh superego and his rebellious id.

When he wasn't performing with all his might and castigating himself for a bad performance, he was acting out his perverse impulses. In one of his first sessions with me, when I asked him what he was thinking, he replied, "Well, what came into my mind was that I feel like jacking off. Oh, Christ, I can't believe I said that."

"What's that about?" I asked.

"I don't know. I guess it would feel good. It would be fun. I'd like to jack off in front of you, and I'd like you to see my dick, see it get hard, and then I'd like you to take your dick out and start whacking off too. I'd like to see your dick, see how it gets hard and what method you use to whack it off, two fingers or whole hand or whatever. Oh, Christ, this is really embarrassing. But I guess I should say all of it. In fact . . . oh, God . . . I'm starting to get hard right now as I'm telling you about this."

This took me a little by surprise. "How would you like me to feel about that?" I asked.

"Honestly? Of course, honestly, stupid," Marvin muttered to himself. "That's what therapy is about. Don't mind me. Anyway, I guess I'd like you to feel excited." He had moved his hand down to his crotch and was rubbing his index finger against it. "Actually, I'd like it if you got a bit of a hard-on right now."

Marvin's id impulses were that of a four-year-old boy whose mother had just caught him masturbating and slapped his hand—a memory that Marvin recalled in one of his sessions. The more a mother rejects a boy's sexuality, the more he is going to assert it. The only change in his behavior is that he will learn to do it in secret and in indirect ways. He will go underground, and his sexuality will become perverse rather than normal.

This happens to quite a number of little boys when they are going through the phallic-narcissistic stage. Psychoanalytic research has shown that nearly all little boys go through this stage, in which they discover their penis and learn that fondling it feels good, and that furthermore penises do magical things such as becoming stiffer and bigger. (Little girls, incidentally, go through a similar vaginal narcissistic stage; however, they seem to suffer even more punitive reactions from parents with regard to their masturbation than boys.) During this phallic-narcissistic stage, little boys become narcissistic about their penises, feeling quite proud of themselves, often going to their mothers or fathers or nannies and displaying themselves and shouting, "Look what I can do!" Of course, this is done in innocence; a four-year-old boy assumes that anything that gives him pleasure and isn't hurting anybody else should be all right to do. Unfortunately, many parents react negatively to such displays, sometimes with subtle frowns, sometimes with a verbal jab ("Don't do that; it's not nice!"), sometimes with a slap, and in extreme cases by an emotional abandonment of the boy, which he experiences as an annihilation of his self. When the boy gets such a negative reaction, he develops a fixation at that stage of development and doesn't move on to mature sexual functioning.

We are referring here to the Oedipal stage of development, a stage to which Freud gave utmost importance but which subsequent psychoanalysts and professionals of other schools have downplayed. Behavioral psychologists, in particular, object to terms such as "Oedipus complex," "phallic-narcissistic stage," and "mature sexual functioning," pointing out that these are subjective terms that can't be scientifically observed or verified. However, Skinner, the father of modern behaviorism, looking at psychodynamics, notes that nearly all of Freud's concepts can be stated in behavioral terms. "Alternate definitions may be derived from the contingencies responsible for the behavior from which the dynamisms are inferred" (1976, p. 171). Thus, most psychoanalytic lingo can generally be restated in behavior terminology: In Marvin's case, he would be said to have experienced adverse conditioning in which he learned to be helpless and to repeat certain behaviors (such as masturbation) that were unwittingly reinforced.

Khan (1979) wrote about the alienation that invariably occurs in perversions. Like Freud, he views what he terms the "paraphiliac" as an id-dominated personality (driven toward the immediate gratification of pleasure) in contrast to the neurotic, who is more of a superego-dominated personality (concerned with moral rectitude). However, the perverse personality, Khan contends, "puts an impersonal object between his desire and his accomplice: this object can be a stereotype fantasy, a gadget or a pornographic image. All three alienate the pervert from himself, as, alas, from the object of his desire" (p. 9). Note that Khan uses the word "accomplice" instead of lover, in order to emphasize that the sexual experience of the pervert consists of his attempting to seduce others into accompanying him in perverse sexuality. In addition, he notes that the pervert is intent on living out fantasies (secondary intimacy) rather than on genuine intimacy between two people who acknowledge each other. Hence, the alienation.

This, basically, was what happened to Marvin, and it explains why Marvin spent so many of his early sessions with me, attempting to persuade me to become his accomplice, and why many of his fantasies were concerned with that theme. In his unconscious mind, the solution to his alienation was to find accomplices; however, no matter how many accomplices he found, he still remained anxious, enraged, and lonely. No matter how many accomplices he found, he still did not have, in Khan's words, a self, and in Freud's, an ego. He treated people as objects rather than as real people, objects to be sexually exploited while he held back his real feelings.

At the beginning of his therapy, Marvin was obsessed with his penis and what it could do. His answer to any stressful situation was to find a closet, a stairway, a bathroom, or a cranny where he could fondle himself. He would masturbate during the daytime when he took his lunch or coffee breaks and at nighttime after his wife went to bed. Masturbation was his life. Sex with others consisted primarily of mutual masturbation. Even when he had sexual intercourse with his wife, he was focused primarily on the masturbatory action of his penis going in and out of his wife's vagina rather than on the overall experience—emotional and physical—of making love.

During the course of his therapy, his masturbation went through various phases. For a year or so, he would masturbate privately in his home or office. Then he began going to sex shops and masturbated in booths while watching straight and gay porn. On occasion he would masturbate while looking at scantily dressed women in glass cages, and sometimes he would call a telephone sex line, usually gay, but sometimes straight. Then there was a time when he went to public restrooms and masturbated with other men. Sometimes he would do it while sitting in a booth, sometimes while standing at the urinal. During this phase, he discovered an underground of men's rooms around the city where young men met and masturbated casually, usually without exchanging a word. One was in a university building; another was in a government building.

As with all people with an obsession, he needed to talk about it, and talk about it he did. Probably around 60 percent of his therapy sessions during the first years of treatment were spent talking about his masturbation. At first he regaled me with elaborate descriptions of his masturbation rites—how often he did it, what techniques he used, how it felt, how big his penis became, how long he was able to maintain erection, how many times he could come. When I neither approved nor disapproved, he became less verbose. Then he began to supply me with a running account of his erotic fantasies.

One of them was a recurring fantasy of meeting up with a witch-woman who scolded him for masturbating and then punished him by having him masturbate for one hour without stopping, which caused his penis to grow larger and larger. This fantasy harked back to a period when his own mother disapproved of his masturbation, and I gave him that interpretation, adding that in the fantasy his mother (the witch), reversed what had happened in childhood by giving him permission to masturbate.

In another fantasy, Marvin imagined himself not as he actually looked but as another man who possessed the kind of large penis, muscular build, and confidence he lacked. As this other man, he would have sex with a woman and satisfy her repeatedly. This fantasy, I told him, compensated for his feelings of masculine inferiority.

Later he had another fantasy in which he would walk around willing other men to masturbate. He had some kind of magical power to control other men's urges in these fantasies, and upon looking at them, they would excuse themselves, run to the nearest bathroom and begin frantically and enjoyably playing with themselves. "I had a fantasy last night that I looked at President Clinton while he was giving a press conference on television," he said one day, "and he suddenly excused himself and had to run to his bedroom to jerk off. I imagined him in the Lincoln bedroom, jerking away at his dick, a smile of glee on his face. Then I imagined that I looked around at you during our session and you pulled out your dick and began whacking it."

"What happened then?" I asked, joining the fantasy.

"I pulled out my dick, and we jerked off together."

"Why does that excite you?"

"Because, deep down I think all men jerk off, but they don't want to admit it."

"Did Bob jerk off?" I asked, referring to his older brother.

"I'm sure he did, but he never admitted it."

"Did your father?"

"God, I don't know. He's so pure. I can't imagine it."

"Do you think I masturbate?"

"I don't know. I hope so."

"What would it mean if you knew that other men masturbated?"

"It would mean I wasn't the only one."

"So you're convinced you're the only man in the world who masturbates?"

"I suppose so. I suppose deep down that's what I really feel. I know it's idiotic. But that's what I feel."

Marvin did not grow up in New York City, but was one of the many who migrate here in search of fame and fortune. His childhood was spent under the glare of the Southern sky. His parents, like many parents, wanted two children, a boy and a girl. They had already had a boy when Marvin was born, and this boy was already his mother's darling and his father's pal. When Marvin popped out of his mother's womb with his infantile penis brazenly quivering, both his parents were apparently disappointed. The older brother became "Mr. Right," and the younger became "Mr. Wrong."

The first and biggest obstacle to his success as an infant was his brother, who did not take kindly to his appearance on the scene. His first memory was of his brother's grinning face peering at him from above the railing of his crib, and a feeling of terror and doom. He had a sense of having been violated somehow by his brother, but no tangible recollection. The second memory was of his mother lying in her bed, too depressed to get up. He was later told—but had no memory of it—that his mother was admitted to a mental hospital several months after his birth.

When a caretaker is depressed, she is unable to properly nurture an infant. As a result, the infant suffers from maternal deprivation. A recent article in the journal *Child Development* (Dawson et al., 1999) reported that infants of depressed mothers exhibit an atypical frontal electrical brain activity during interactions with their mother and with others. The writers noted that reduced left frontal brain activity is indicative of diminished positive emotions. This research confirms earlier studies by Spitz (1965) and Bowlby (1979) with orphaned infants. Their studies showed to what extent maternal deprivation affects an infant's emotional development. Infants can die from deprivation, contracting a malady called marasmus, becoming so depressed that they lose their will to live. Spitz observed that about 30 percent of orphans in a foundling hospital during World War II, given only brief feedings by a succession of nurses, developed this disorder. Marvin didn't die, but he suffered much damage to his ego: his self-confidence, self-esteem, perception of reality, and ability to cope were all severely hampered.

His mother, perhaps out of her disappointment at not begetting a girl child, was, in addition to being depressed, impatient with Marvin, particularly with his developing masculinity. He remembered how, during toilet training, she would put him on the toilet roughly and order him to move his bowels, leaving him all alone to fend for himself. Once she caught him playing with his penis while he was on the potty. He smiled at her, held up his organ, and said, "Mommy, touch my penis!"

"Don't talk like that; that's dirty!" she replied, pulling his hand away from the offending appendage.

"But it's *my* penis."

"Shush!"

"Mine! Mine! Mine!"

"I said shush!"

On other occasions she would slap his hand and tell him he was being naughty.

Not only did he have to contend with these rebukes from his mother, but he also had to parry more direct attacks from his brother. Since his mother was depressed much of the time and therefore unable to function, Marvin was left unprotected from this brother. Marvin recalled that Bob waged an all-out "campaign of terror" every day when he came home from school. Not only would he physically batter Marvin, but also he would psychologically castrate him. At times he would pretend to be Marvin's friend, leading him to believe that he was going to be nice to him; but the moment Marvin started to believe it, Bob would flip into "the monster voice and the monster laugh" and would betray Marvin in some way, cackling and calling him an idiot.

He wanted to scream. He wanted to do much more than scream. He wanted to smash in his brother's face. He did not know why his brother hated him so much or why his mother and father seemed to ignore him. All he knew was that there was nothing much he could do about any of it. He couldn't retaliate because his brother would beat him up, nor could he scream, because that would only make his mother irritated, and if his mother became irritated, his father would come to her aid and tell both boys to shut up. "You know your mother can't stand screaming!"

Indeed, the mother and brother often seemed to be in cahoots against Marvin when, at the age of five, he put on his underwear backward, and his brother pointed at him and laughed. "Mom, come look at Marvy. He's got his underwear on backward." His mother shook her head and joined her favorite son in his merry derision.

"So he does."

"He doesn't know his front from his behind."

"I do too," Marvin fiercely defended himself.

"No you don't."

"I do, I do, I do!"

Feeling that his masculinity, his sexuality, and his very being were constantly under attack by his brother and mother, Marvin turned to his father as if he were a lifebuoy in a turbulent sea. He needed desperately to talk to somebody about the confused thoughts and feelings swirling inside him. However, his father was not there for him either. He abdicated all authority with regard to family matters to his wife. A passive male, he wished to avoid confrontation at all costs, and in particular to avoid his wife's hysteria. Therefore, he would not intervene on Marvin's behalf. Moreover, his father was a silent, pious man, a deacon in the church, a stockbroker, who did not have time for the petty domestic concerns of the household. Instead of helping Marvin, he made matters worse by insisting on walking around the house naked each night after he had taken his shower, brandishing his huge carotene penis like some kind of emblem of supremacy.

"Dad?" Marvin would venture, sitting beside his naked father as the latter read *The Wall Street Journal,* oblivious to the hypnotic emanations of his reproductive organ, which dwarfed Marvin's own meager nodule. "Yes, Marvin. What is it? Oh, my God, IBM went up six and a half points!"

"That's great. Dad, could I ask you something?"

"Of course, son. And look at this. Will you look at this? Goodyear is up ten points! Ten!"

"Dad?"

"Yes, yes, yes. What is it?"

"Never mind."

During latency, he forgot about his penis and began to eat. He became the fat boy that his schoolmates loved to tease. By adolescence he had become a loner. More than anything else, he liked to ensconce himself in his basement bedroom, where he would masturbate and eat chocolate chip cookies to his heart's content. Alone in his "bunker," he could imagine things. He could imagine being a handsome movie star with the most magnificent genitals in the world. He could imagine many women and men admiring him. He could imagine coming home to Alabama as a celebrity, sitting down to dinner with his family, his older brother apologizing to him, and his parents begging his forgiveness.

Such family triumph fantasies are common among artists, and some artists have the feeling that these kinds of revenge fantasies fuel their creative impulse and drive them toward success. However, as I pointed out earlier, these fantasies seem in fact to be generally destructive because their obsessive nature keeps artists mired in an art-as-revenge mode. Hence, creativity doesn't flow naturally and the view portrayed by the artist (if he or she is a writer) is colored by anger rather than being properly transformed into a vehicle of entertainment and enlightenment. Obsessed by fantasies of revenge, the artist puts pressure on the creative process, for it must now somehow manage to serve to resurrect the artist's lost self and all that this entails: namely, the sense that it is all right to be alive and that he or she is a worthwhile and lovable human being. If the artist does achieve success, he or she quickly realizes that revenge is not sweet, but empty. No amount of success can bring back the self-esteem, confidence, and coping ability that was not acquired in early childhood, and no amount of belated admiration by family members can make up for neglect during the early years. For this reason, success is often followed by depression and a flight to alcoholism, drugs, and sexual escapism, as a means of handling the emptiness.

Marvin's therapy could be divided into three phases. The first phase, which might be called the narcissistic phase, lasted about two years. During this phase, all I tried to do was provide a safe environment in which Marvin could verbalize all his perverse impulses and not be punished for it (reversing what had happened in his family milieu). The second phase, during which I used primarily behavioral techniques, lasted about three more years. A third, psychodynamic phase, went on for another several years after that.

The behavioral therapy phase began when he came in one day and did not talk about masturbation. He continued not to talk about it for a few weeks, which was quite unusual. Finally, toward the middle of the session, he brought it up.

"I've been deliberately not talking about masturbation for the last few sessions," he said. "Have you noticed?"

"I noticed. Why?"

"Because I just wanted to see if I could do it. It occurred to me that there has hardly been a session in the last three years when I haven't talked about it."

"That's true."

"And anyway I've been feeling lately—well, actually for some time now, or for a while, or whatever you call a few months, I guess a few months could be said to be some time, couldn't it? GET ON WITH IT, MARVIN! God! Blablablablabla! All right, I can say this. I really can." He shook his head rapidly as though trying to throw off the bad synapses dwelling inside and jamming up the works, then proceeded to demonstrate that he had begun to look at himself with more objectivity. He related that he had started to worry about how much he was masturbating and the kinds of risks he was taking—frequenting sleazy public places such as porn shops and rest rooms where he could get caught. He had also begun to fear that he might catch a disease such as AIDS, although he knew from a rational standpoint that one could not catch AIDS via mutual masturbation. He was concerned about cheating on his wife, and dreaded the possibility of his wife or mother finding out about such activities. Finally, he didn't like the way the excessive masturbation was making him feel. "It's getting to the point where I'm starting to feel weird, creepy. My life isn't measured in coffee spoons, but in dicks. My dick, other guys' dicks. Dicks, dicks, dicks. Help!"

I realized he was now ready for help in gaining control over his acting out. Therefore, I took great pains to explain a behavioral intervention that I had borrowed from Milton Erickson—a paradoxical technique that plugged into his fantasies. Although I am a psychoanalyst, I often use other modalities if and when necessary, and it is often necessary. Psychoanalytic therapy works well only with some people, and then only at a certain point in the treatment. It doesn't work well with addictive personalities, for example, until such time as they have overcome their addictions. Marvin's masturbation was not normal masturbation but an addiction—one to which he had now admitted (the first step in an addict's recovery).

His recurring sexual fantasy about the witch-mother who ordered him to masturbate represented a wish and a clue regarding the treatment. Understanding this not only helped me to figure Marvin out but also provided me with a method. He had become fixated and obsessed with masturbation because he had not been given the response he needed at a certain phase of development. To resolve this fixation, I determined to provide him with the antidote to this repudiation—playing the "witch" who would give him permission to enjoy his infantile sexuality. I did not say this to him, but instead simply explained that I was using a behavioral program.

I told him he was to listen very carefully to my instructions and to follow them to the letter. I asked him if he would be willing to do that. He said he would. I repeated this first instruction several times and then said that beginning the following Monday I wanted him to masturbate ten hours a week and write down when, where, and how long he masturbated and how many orgasms he had when he did so. I asked him to note the quality of his erections (semi-hard, hard, rock hard) and the length of his orgasms in approximate seconds. I wanted to know the nature of his ejaculation—did it squirt out or seep out—and the volume of the semen (slight, average, heavy).

He gulped, "Really," but his cheeks were flushed, and I could tell he was excited by the prospect.

I repeated these instructions again and again in different words. I told him that if he did not think he could do the ten hours, then we should forget the plan, because the plan would only work if he did it exactly as presented. I warned him that he would think of many reasons not to do the plan. It might seem to be fun at first, but eventually he would get tired of it and try to find excuses to stop. But if he stopped, the entire plan would be for naught, and he would be even worse off than before because he would hate himself for not being able to carry through with it. I said I did not want to start the plan unless I had his absolute assurance that he would not quit under any circumstances. I said again that it would be the hardest thing he had ever done but guaranteed him that if he did it, he would definitely overcome his obsession with masturbation and feel much better about himself. I said his self-esteem would increase dramatically if he succeeded.

I went on for almost the entire session, speaking in a monotone and repeating everything several times so that the words would be as hypnotic as possible. I threw in a lengthy interpretation about why he masturbated—how it served both as an act of rebellion against society (which symbolized his parents) and as a boost to his masculinity. Finally, I reassured him over and over that it was all right for him to have a penis and to do with it whatever he wanted, so long as it didn't interfere with his life or other people's lives. He listened quite intently to my explanation, more intently than he had ever listened before. At the end, I asked, "Well, how does it sound?"

"It sounds like it would be fun!" he blurted out. "I can't wait to start. I'll probably go somewhere and whack off as soon as I leave."

"Go forth and masturbate," I replied.

After the first week, he came back beaming excitedly. "It was great. I had permission to do what I love to do." His notes about his masturbation, giving details of all aspects of his practices as I had instructed, were copious.

After the second week, he came back sighing. "It was getting a little bit tiring this week. I wanted to stop in the middle of the week because my dick was sore, and I was feeling a bit self-conscious. Also, I must confess I was a tad resentful toward you." His notes were less copious.

After the third week, he came back wincing. He had no notes. "I'm extremely angry at myself," he said, lying stiffly on the couch. "As you've probably realized, I couldn't finish. I stopped the program last Wednesday. So shoot me!"

"Why are you angry at yourself?"

"Because I'm a failure. I couldn't do it."

"Why aren't you angry at me?" I asked. "I'm the one who gave you an impossible task."

"As a matter of fact, I am angry at you."

"Tell me about it."

He did, and the therapy took a sharp turn for the better. His masturbation had become a job rather than a joy, an act of duty rather than of rebellion. The anger that had been acted out in this obsessive act now came to the surface and was directed at its source—his mother, father, and brother—and at me in the transference. Once I had accepted it and had analyzed it, a new, more authentically emotional bond began to form between us. This led directly into the third phase of the treatment—the psychodynamic phase. Whereas the previous phase was spent focusing almost entirely on symptoms, this phase was devoted to reconstructing what happened in his childhood, how it affected his present life, and how it was being played out in the transference relationship. It was during this phase that Marvin worked through the feelings that underlay his symptoms.

There came a turning point in Marvin's treatment when he suddenly got in touch with his core feelings. Most of the time people in therapy never discover these core feelings; they are too painful and are too buried beneath layers of repression. Marvin had gone on for several years keeping me and his real self (his core feelings) at a distance. On the surface he was the dutiful patient, but beneath the surface he was quietly rebelling, and there was never even an inkling of any real emotion. One day all that changed. It happened at around the time I put him into a therapy group.

He had started out in the group the same way he had started out in his individual treatment, by attempting to seduce the members of the group into being his accomplices. When they responded by neither rebuking his seductions nor accepting them, but instead expressing thoughts about the loneliness they were picking up in his manner, he was forced to take a look at that.

His participation in the group pushed his individual therapy to a new, deeper level. One day, in an individual session, he began to cry for the first time. He had been talking about the time after his mother came home from the mental hospital. This was during his infancy and young childhood. For several years after returning from the hospital, she was apparently in a state of depression, as I noted earlier, and was not able to properly nurture her children. During these years Marvin felt abandoned by his mother and persecuted by his older brother. As he talked about this period of time, his face wrinkled up like a prune and his voice began to waver.

"Oh, God, oh God! Oh, please, please God!" Marvin exclaimed, and he let out one of the loudest screams I have ever hard. It was an angry, half scream and half cry—the kind of cry one hears from infants and preschoolers. He had regressed, emotionally, to the time he was remembering. "I'm so afraid. I'm so, so terrified," he said, and let out another scream.

"Why are you terrified?" I asked.

"Because of him. Because of Bob. I'm so afraid. Every day I'm so afraid. I dread the time when he comes home from school. Even when he's not home, I can't relax. I could never relax. I still can't. Oh, God!" He began to sob.

"What happens when he comes home from school?"

"Oh, God. I don't want to remember this! He'll hit me. He'll mock me. He'll laugh at me. He'll beat me up. He'll tell me that I'm an idiot. He'll tell me that Mom's sickness is my fault. He'll tell me he wishes I were never born. Oh, God, I was at his mercy. There was nobody around."

"Where was your mother?"

"In bed."

"What would she say?"

"She'd just yell out if we were noisy."

"She'd tell you both to be quiet. But she'd never tell Bob to leave you alone."

"Never. Oh, God. Oh, God!" He let out another scream and cried for a few minutes in an angry, regressive manner, then stopped himself. I had the sense of two people lying there on the couch: one, a very young and an extremely hurt little boy; the other, an adult man struggling to restrain the little boy's cry.

"What would you like to say to your mother? Tell her what you need from her."

"Mommy, I need your love!" he cried out angrily and broke into deep sobbing. "Oh, Mommy, I need your love so much."

Once he had made this first breakthrough, he continued to go to this cathartic place almost every session for several months, both in individual and group sessions. Being able to cry and be vulnerable in the group sessions was perhaps even more important than his being able to do so in his individual sessions; the group became the supportive family environment he had lacked in childhood and hence served a reparative function. Eventually the intensity of his anger diminished and he journeyed to the cathartic place less often. After the first few months, there followed several years in which he would alternately go back to that place and then soberly spend a few sessions analyzing how his traumatic childhood and the core feelings he had been repressing were affecting his present life and, in particular, his creative pursuits. He gradually understood why he was blocked and how to get unblocked: that is, he understood the process of letting go of past hurts and truly living in the present.

As he worked through these core feelings and integrated them into his life, he became more authentic in the group and in his individual sessions. For a time, the people in the group became the most important people in his life, more important than his parents, his wife, and his best friends. He kept track of all their birthdays, anniversaries, and even the birthdays of their children. He often spoke of how much he loved them and appreciated them. In his individual sessions, he expressed similar sentiments to me. Meanwhile his artistic career was on the rebound.

At a certain point he started to write humorous one-act plays. These plays, like his fantasies, were a bit on the perverse side, but he had managed to "regress in the service of the ego" as Kris (1952) put it. That is, whereas before his id had dominated his ego, now his ego controlled his id, and in order to allow his creativity to flow, his ego allowed his id a kind of creative free reign. This free rein entailed a regression to a childlike state in which imagination could spring forth uninhibited by adult restraints. However, his adult ego made sure that the writings that resulted were not simply indulgences but were modified by an objective adult sensibility.

One of those one-act plays, *The Masturbators,* had a theme that was very similar to one of the themes prominent in his early fantasies. In it, a mother catches her adolescent son masturbating. She begins to scorn him, but he stops her and demands to know if she has ever masturbated. At first she vehemently denies it. But eventually, after a lengthy, humorous interrogation by her son (he questions her in the manner of an FBI agent), she confesses, and then grins coyly as she recalls her first masturbation. At that moment, the father and brother enter the house and the son similarly begins to interrogate the father and brother. After a while they too confess. Next the sister enters and is likewise forced to confess, and finally, the grandmother. In the end, the adolescent protagonist suggests that they all "adjourn to the bedroom" for a family masturbation session, noting that, "A family that sprays together stays together." All of this was quite hilarious and was a wonderful spoof of family hypocrisy.

It was apparent in this and other plays how Marvin was now able to sublimate his core feelings about his family and transform those feelings into something that had meaning beyond his individual conflicts—which is the essence of art. By writing a play about a family that symbolized his own, he could objectify conflicts that he had formerly internalized. This was both therapeutic and illuminating: an indication of how far he had come in terms of strengthening his ego: elevating his self-confidence, elevating his self-esteem, and improving his all-around functioning.

In contrast to his early sessions, in which I was merely an object to be seduced, in his later sessions I became a beloved mentor whose "visits" he cherished. He often came to his sessions beaming as he strutted through the door.

"I feel great! I just got another play accepted. It's just a loft theater, but it's a start." Formerly, he had not allowed himself to feel great. In his head, the voice of his brother would mock him and tell him to stop acting like an idiot. But now, because of his therapy work, that voice had all but gone away, and he could openly verbalize to me that he felt great and get the appropriate response from me—acceptance of his feelings.

"That's nice," I said. "You've worked hard, and you deserve to feel great. That's a good feeling."

"Yes, it is. And I owe it to you and to the group."

"And to your own hard work."

"I'll take some credit. I can do that. You know, I feel like giving you a big hug right now."

"I feel like giving you one back."

We hugged each other symbolically.

Marvin's playwriting career continued to progress. Eventually he wrote and directed a full-length play at an off-off Broadway theater in the East Village. It was another slightly perverse, but quite imaginative comedy. The group and I went together to see the play and, naturally, saw meanings in it that the other members of the audience could not see. Afterward we all met Marvin backstage.

"Bravo," one group member said. "I really feel proud of you. And also a little jealous."

"You've come a long way, baby," another said.

"Yes," Marvin replied, sparkling in that special way theater people do on a successful first night. "And now I'm going to bring all of you with me."

From that point on Marvin became sort of the "group whip," encouraging others to follow his lead in getting in touch with their deepest layer of feelings and working through them. It was a good lead to follow.

Appendix

Tests of Inhibited Creativity

The following tests have been designed to detect various aspects of personality that are associated with creativity. Test 1 is a straightforward questionnaire that examines the cognitive elements generally found in the thinking of people who are blocked emotionally and inhibited in their creativity. Test 2 is a visual test that exams a person's creative ideas. Test 3 is a projective test, a variation of the TAT that psychologists use, except that in this case only one drawing is used and the aim is slightly different. Test 4 is a personality test, aimed at detecting psychopathology that may typically underpin blocked creativity.

These tests may be administered by a psychotherapist, or readers may take them on their own. Test takers are encouraged to be completely honest in answering the questionnaires; otherwise the tests will be invalid. The questionnaires have no time limit, but the other two tests have limits that must be strictly enforced. The entire battery shouldn't take more than one hour. The answers to all four tests are at the end of this appendix. (No cheating.)

Good luck!

INHIBITED CREATIVITY TEST 1

Instructions: Please answer these questions as truthfully as possible. If you cannot answer "Always" or "Never" then the answer is probably "Sometimes." There is no time limit.

1. When I start to do something creative, such as writing, painting, or composing, I start comparing myself to others and then I lose interest.
   Always___ Sometimes___ Never___

2. When I engage in a creative project, I am not satisfied with it because it is generally not perfect enough, and so I give up.
   Always___ Sometimes___ Never___

3. When I engage in a creative project, I have fantasies of being rich, famous, or returning home to my family in triumph.
   Always___ Sometimes___ Never___

4. When I engage in a creative project, I am not thinking about anything else except the fun of the project.
   Always___ Sometimes___ Never___

5. I do not care if anybody else understands my art, as long as I understand it.
   Always___ Sometimes___ Never___

6. Whenever I engage in a creative project, I start thinking about all the books (paintings, compositions, etc.) that already exist, and I tell myself, "Oh, well, that's already been done. What's the use?"
   Always___ Sometimes___ Never___

7. I'd like to do something creative, but I can never find the time to do it.
   Always___ Sometimes___ Never___

8. Whenever I did something creative as a child, my parents always said something like, "That's nice, but if you want to make money, you should go into a profession or business."
   Always___ Sometimes___ Never___

9. I do not have any problems doing my art (writing, composition, etc.), but I shudder when I think of trying to sell it.
   Always___ Sometimes___ Never___

10. People keep telling me I should change this or that about my paintings (writing, compositions), but I do not listen to them. I hate criticism, and anyway, only I know what is best for my work.

     Always___ Sometimes___ Never___

11. Whenever I am trying to write/paint/practice, I think about other things I would like to do, such as playing tennis or cleaning the house or going to the beach.

     Always___ Sometimes___ Never___

12. It is hard for me to be alone with myself.

     Always___ Sometimes___ Never___

13. I am afraid that if I create something that is really great some people will be jealous.

     Always___ Sometimes___ Never___

14. I find myself constantly having fantasies about fame, even when I am trying to create.

     Always___ Sometimes___ Never___

15. Whenever I do something artistic, I always think it is childish and that I need to grow up and do adult work.

     Always___ Sometimes___ Never___

INHIBITED CREATIVITY TEST 2

Instructions: On the following page you will find a series of squares. In each square is a printed line or lines. Use these as a basis for a separate, original drawing of something recognizable. Work quickly and do not bother with details or with artistic technique. Be concerned with ideas, not technique. Time limit: 5 minutes.

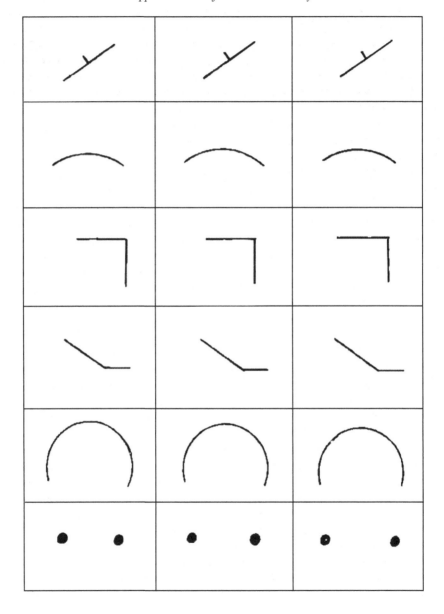

INHIBITED CREATIVITY TEST 3

Instructions: On the following page is a drawing. Study the drawing. Then create a story about what you think is happening, has happened, or will happen in the drawing. Make up more than one story if you like. You can write the story or stories below or on a separate page. Time limit: 10 minutes.

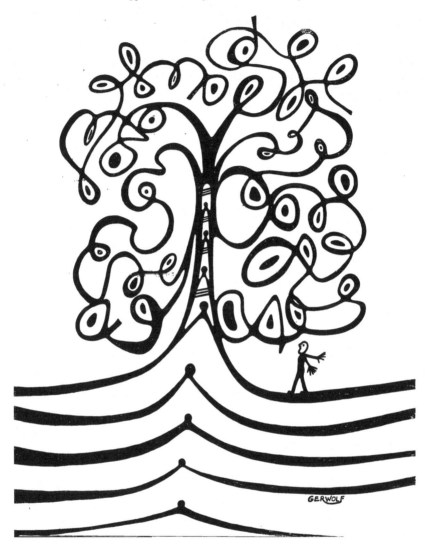

INHIBITED CREATIVITY TEST 4

Instructions: Please answer the following questions as honestly as you can. If you try to give the "right" answers, this test will be useless. Although there is no time limit, go through the questions quickly without thinking too much about them.

1. I spend days thinking about situations that have felt humiliating.

   Always___ Sometimes___ Never___

2. I have trouble getting to sleep at night.

   Always___ Sometimes___ Never___

3. I wake up early and then cannot get back to sleep.

   Always___ Sometimes___ Never___

4. Whenever somebody says something hurtful to me, it takes me a few days before I realize I am hurt.

   Always___ Sometimes___ Never___

5. I find myself feeling terrified of certain things or situations that do not seem to bother others.

   Always___ Sometimes___ Never___

6. I find myself feeling happy or sad or angry without knowing exactly why I feel that way.

   Always___ Sometimes___ Never___

7. I have the feeling my work is not going to be as good as other people's work, no matter what I do.

   Always___ Sometimes___ Never___

8. I do not get the respect from people that I deserve, but others get much more than they deserve.

   Always___ Sometimes___ Never___

9. I am unhappy with the way my life is going, but I don't know what to do about it.

   Always___ Sometimes___ Never___

10. I do not feel quite myself unless I've had a drink, smoked some marijuana, or taken some other drug.

    Always___ Sometimes___ Never___

11. I get really upset when somebody I know fails to greet me when we pass on the street.

        Always___   Sometimes___   Never___

12. Most people do not like me because they are jealous or resentful of me.

        Always___   Sometimes___   Never___

13. People keep telling me I am oversensitive, but I think they just do not want to admit their own cruelty.

        Always___   Sometimes___   Never___

14. I think that life is very unfair because inevitably the wrong people get ahead.

        Always___   Sometimes___   Never___

15. I feel mistreated by people, and I want to hurt them.

        Always___   Sometimes___   Never___

ANSWERS

Inhibited Creativity Test 1

The questions in this test address the common symptoms of being blocked. If you answer "Always" to seven or more of them, "Sometimes" to ten or more of them, consider yourself fairly blocked.

Inhibited Creative Test 2

In this test, give yourself one point for each separate recognizable drawing. There are eighteen squares on the test, so a perfect score is eighteen. In general, points are given for the variety of ideas. If you use the same idea two or more times (for example, if there is more than one human face), you get no points for the second or third face, unless they are in some way quite different from the other face. Naturally, squares left undrawn get no points. If your score is 12 or higher, your creativity is flowing. If your score is 15 or higher, it's streaming.

Uninhibited Creativity Test 3

The aim of this test is to create as many imaginative stories as possible based on the drawing. The more detailed, surprising, exciting, or humorous the stories are, the higher your score. Scoring this test is a bit complex, and readers who take it may want to have a friend help them to determine the extent of creativity in the stories. On the other hand, if you have trouble thinking of stories, or if you can only think of one brief story, this would be an indication of a block. In addition, if you create more than one story, take note of the prevalent themes. For example, is there a lot of aggression? Violence? Sexuality? This might tell you something about your unconscious conflicts.

Uninhibited Creativity Test 4

This test is a test of psychopathology—that is, of how neurotic you are. Since neurosis often impedes creativity, it is an important contributor to creative blocks. If you answer "Always" to seven or more of the questions, or "Sometimes" to ten or more, consider yourself fairly blocked.

If all four tests indicate that you are blocked, you might want to consider seeking professional help. Think of it as hiring a personal coach or trainer. A good therapist, like a good coach, can help you get to that next level in art and life.

References

Alexander, F. (1953). The psychoanalyst looks at contemporary art. In W. Philips (Ed.), *Art and Psychoanalysis* (pp. 346-368). Cleveland: Meridian Books, 1963.

Bergler, E. (1945). On a five-layer structure in sublimation. *The Psychoanalytic Quarterly,* 14:76-97.

Bonaparte, M. (1949). *The Life and Works of Edgar Allen Poe.* London: Imago Publishing Company.

Bowlby, J. (1979). *The Making and Breaking of Affectional Bonds.* London: Tavistock.

Dawson, G., Frey, K., Panagiodes, H., Yamada, E. (1999). Left frontal brain electrical activity in infants of depressed mothers. *Child Development,* 70:1058-1066.

Deutsch, H. (1942). Some forms of emotional disturbance and their relationship to schizophrenia. *Psychoanalytic Quarterly,* 11:301-321.

Epstein, L. and Feiner, A. H. (1979). *Countertransference: The Therapist's Contribution to the Therapeutic Situation.* Northvale, NJ: Aronson.

Freud, S. (1905). Jokes and their relation to the unconscious. *The Complete Psychological Works of Sigmund Freud,* 8:3-238, New York: W. W. Norton.

_____ (1907). Delusions and dreams in Jensen's Gradiva. *The Complete Psychological Works of Sigmund Freud,* 9:3-95, New York: W. W. Norton.

_____ (1908a). Character and anal eroticism. *The Complete Psychological Works of Sigmund Freud,* 9:167-176, New York: W. W. Norton.

_____ (1908b). Creative writers and daydreaming. *The Complete Psychological Works of Sigmund Freud,* 9:142-153, New York: W. W. Norton.

_____ (1910). Leonardo da Vinci and a memory of his childhood. *The Complete Psychological Works of Sigmund Freud,* 10:3-152, New York: W. W. Norton.

_____ (1911). Formulations on two principles of mental functioning. *The Complete Psychological Works of Sigmund Freud,* 12:215-226, New York: W. W. Norton.

_____ (1915). Observations on transference-love. *The Complete Psychological Works of Sigmund Freud,* 12:157-174, New York: W. W. Norton.

Goodwin, F. K. and Jamison, K. R. (1990). *Manic-Depressive Illness.* New York: Oxford University Press.

Greenacre, P. (1971). *Emotional Growth,* Volume 2. New York: International Universities Press.

Jacobson, E. (1971). *Depression: Comparative Studies of Normal, Neurotic, and Psychotic Conditions.* New York: International Universities Press.

Kernberg, O. E., Selzer, M. A., Koenigsberg, H. W. (1989). *Psychodynamic Psychotherapy with Borderline Patients.* New York: Basic Books.

129

Khan, M. M. R. (1979). *Alienation in the Perversions*. New York: International Universities Press.

Kohut, H. (1971). *The Analysis of the Self*. New York: International Universities Press.

Kris, E. (1952). Psychoanalysis and the study of creative imagination. In L. M. Newman (Ed.), *Selected Papers of Ernst Kris* (pp. 473-493). New Haven: Yale University Press.

Lacan, J. (1982). *Feminine Sexuality*. Juliet Mitchell and Jacqueline Rose (Eds.). New York: W. W. Norton.

Ludwig, A. (1996). *The Price of Greatness*. New York: Guilford Press.

Mahler, M. S., Pine, F., Bergman, A. (1975). *The Psychological Birth of the Infant*. London: Maresfield Library.

Margolis, B. D. (1987). Treatment and transition: Observation on modern psychoanalysis. *Modern Psychoanalysis, 12*:163-178.

Marshall, R. J. (1979). Countertransference with children and adolescents. In L. Epstein and A. H. Feiner (Eds.), *Countertransference: The Therapist's Contribution to the Therapeutic Situation*. Northvale, NJ: Aronson.

May, R. (1975). *The Courage to Create*. New York: W. W. Norton.

Meadow, P. (1987). The myth of the impersonal analyst. *Modern Psychoanalysis, 12*:131-150.

Miller, A. (1983). *For Your Own Good: Hidden Cruelty in Childhood and the Roots of Violence*. New York: Farrar, Straus, Giroux.

Niederland, W. G. (1967). Clinical aspects of creativity. *American Imago, 20*:6-33.

Offit, S. (1998). What Is Psychoanalysis? A brochure by the National Association for the Advancement of Psychoanalysis.

Philips, W. (1957). *Art and Psychoanalysis*. Cleveland: Meridian Books.

Rank, O. (1932). *Art and Artist*. New York: Knopf.

Reich, W. (1933). *Character Analysis,* Third Edition. Translated by U. R. Carfagno. New York: Pocket Books, 1973.

Rose, O. (1980). Some aspects of aesthetics in the light of the rapprochement subphase. In R. F. Lax, S. Bach, and J. A. Barland (Eds.), *Rapprochement: The Critical Subphase of Separation/Individuation* (pp. 112-126). New York: Aronson.

Rosen, J. (1962). *Direct Psychoanalytic Psychiatry*. New York: Grune and Stratton.

Salinger, J. D. (1951). *The Catcher in the Rye*. Boston: Little, Brown and Company.

_____ (1953). *Nine Stories*. Boston: Little, Brown and Company.

_____ (1961). *Franny and Zooey*. Boston: Little, Brown and Company.

_____ (1963). *Raise High the Roof Beam, Carpenters, and Seymour: An Introduction*. Boston: Little, Brown and Company.

Salinger, M. (2000). *Dream Catcher*. New York: Pocket Books.

Schoenewolf, G. (1993). *Counterresistance: The Therapist's Interference with the Therapeutic Process*. Northvale, NJ: Aronson.

_____ (1996). Soiling and the anal-narcissistic character. *American Journal of Psychoanalysis, 57*:47-62.

Seligman, M. E. P. (1992). *Helplessness: On Depression, Development, and Death.* New York: Knopf.

Shengold, L. (1979). Child abuse and deprivation: Soul murder. *Journal of the American Psychoanalytic Association,* 17:533-560.

_____ (1989). *Halo in the Sky.* New Haven: Yale University Press.

Skinner, B. F. (1976). *About Behaviorism.* New York: Vintage Books.

Spitz, R. A. (1965). *The First Year of Life: A Psychoanalytic Study of Normal and Deviant Development of Object Relations.* New York: International Universities Press.

Spotnitz, H. (1976). *Psychotherapy of Preoedipal Conditions.* Northvale, NJ: Aronson.

_____ (1985). *Modern Psychoanalysis of the Schizophrenic Patient,* Second Edition. New York: Human Sciences Press.

Winnicott, D. W. (1947). Hate in the countertransference. In *Through Paediatrics to Psycho-Analysis* (pp. 194-203). New York: Basic Books, 1975.

_____ (1965). *The Family and Individual Development.* London: Tavistock.

Index

NOTES FOR PROFESSIONAL LIBRARIANS
AND LIBRARY USERS

This is an original book title published by The Haworth Clinical Practice Press, an imprint of The Haworth Press, Inc. Unless otherwise noted in specific chapters with attribution, materials in this book have not been previously published elsewhere in any format or language.

CONSERVATION AND PRESERVATION NOTES

Printed in the United States
by Baker & Taylor Publisher Services